ADHD MANAGEMENT IN KIDS

A Kid's Journey to ADHD Success

Peggy S. Ortiz

Table of Contents

Introduction

Understanding ADHD in Children

ADHD, or Consideration Shortfall/Hyperactivity Problem, is a neurodevelopmental problem that usually shows up in youth and can persevere into adulthood. It's portrayed by side effects like absentmindedness, hyperactivity, and impulsivity.

Heedlessness: Kids with ADHD might experience issues remaining on track, adhering to directions, arranging undertakings, and frequently committing indiscreet errors.

Hyperactivity: They might be unnecessarily dynamic, nervous, and experience difficulty standing by, even in circumstances where it's normal.

Impulsivity: Kids with ADHD might act automatically, hinder others, and experience issues hanging tight.

Analysis ordinarily includes noticing these ways of behaving after some time and taking into account their effect on day-to-day existence. Treatment choices can incorporate social treatment, prescription, and backing from teachers and guardians to assist with overseeing side effects and further develop a youngster's working. Early intercession is critical for better long-haul results.

Assuming that you have explicit inquiries or need more data, go ahead and inquire.

Kinds of ADHD:

There are three subtypes of ADHD:

Overwhelmingly Distracted Show: Described mostly by troubles with consideration and association.

Overwhelmingly Hyperactive-Imprudent Show: Described mostly by hyperactivity and impulsivity.

Joined Show: Includes a blend of both carelessness and hyperactivity-impulsivity side effects, which is the most widely recognized subtype.

Reasons for ADHD:

While the specific reason is obscure, ADHD is accepted to result from a blend of hereditary, neurological, and ecological variables. It's not brought about by poor nurturing or a lot of sugar, as certain misguided judgments propose.

Side effects and Effect:

Side effects can shift in seriousness, and not all kids with ADHD will show similar ways of behaving.

Untreated ADHD can influence a youngster's scholarly exhibition, connections, confidence, and generally personal satisfaction.

Treatment and the Board:

Conduct treatment: This incorporates techniques to further develop conduct, discretion, and association.

Prescription: Energizer meds (e.g., methylphenidate, amphetamine) and non-energizer drugs can assist with overseeing side effects.

Instructive help: custom curriculum administrations and study hall facilities can be useful.

Parental contribution: Guardians can learn strategies to all the more likely help their youngster and establish an organized climate.

Long haul Viewpoint:

With suitable treatment and backing, numerous youngsters with ADHD can have fruitful existences. Early intercession and a far-reaching treatment plan customized to the youngster's requirements are fundamental.

It's essential to talk with medical services experts, like pediatricians, clinicians, or specialists, for a legitimate assessment and direction if you suspect your kid might have ADHD. They can give a determination and assist with making an individualized arrangement for dealing with the condition.

What is ADHD?

ADHD represents Attention Deficit Hyperactivity Disorder. It's a neurodevelopmental problem that influences the two youngsters and grown-ups. Individuals with ADHD might experience issues with consideration, motivation control, and hyperactivity. Side effects can incorporate carelessness, fretfulness, trouble remaining on track, and rashness. ADHD can influence different parts of an individual's life, including school, work, and connections. Treatment choices frequently incorporate treatment, prescription, or a mix of both. It's fundamental to talk with a medical services professional for a legitimate conclusion and customized therapy plan on the off chance that you suspect you or somebody you know has ADHD.

Common Symptoms in Kids

Normal ADHD side effects in children can include:

Distractedness: Trouble zeroing in on errands, committing imprudent errors, carelessness, and inconvenience sorting out exercises.

Hyperactivity: Anxiety, unnecessary talking, and squirming.

Impulsivity: Interfering with others, trouble standing by, and pursuing rash choices.

Trouble with association: Chaotic rooms or things, inconvenience adhering to guidelines, and distraction.

Distraction: Carelessness in day-to-day exercises, for example, neglecting to do schoolwork, errands, or carrying important things to school.

Trouble in school: Battles with errands that require supported consideration, such as paying attention to addresses or finishing tasks, and frequently committing reckless errors.

The trouble with the association: Inconvenience keeping their assets and school materials coordinated, frequently losing things like books, pencils, or toys.

Unfortunate using time effectively: Trouble assessing time, prompting issues with being reliable or overseeing time proficiently.

Debilitated interactive abilities: Trouble in shaping and keeping up with companionships because of imprudent ways of behaving or inconvenience in perceiving meaningful gestures.

Close-to-home dysregulation: Emotional episodes, uplifted profound responses, and trouble overseeing dissatisfaction or outrage.

It's memorable that these side effects can differ in force and show among kids with ADHD. Finding and treatment ought to be completed by a certified medical services professional.

Diagnosis and Assessment

ADHD, or Consideration Shortage/Hyperactivity Problem, is regularly analyzed through a far-reaching evaluation process. Here are the key advances included:

Clinical Assessment: A proficient medical care proficient, like a specialist or pediatrician, directs an intensive clinical assessment. They gather data about the singular's clinical and mental history, as well as their ongoing side effects.

Side effect Appraisal: ADHD is portrayed by side effects like absentmindedness, hyperactivity, and impulsivity. The clinician surveys the presence and seriousness of these side effects, frequently utilizing normalized rating scales.

Preclude Different Circumstances: It's vital to preclude other clinical or mental circumstances that could mirror ADHD side effects. These may incorporate learning handicaps, nervousness problems, or state of mind issues.

Gathering Data: Data from guardians, educators, or different parental figures is significant, particularly for evaluating side effects across various settings and settings.

DSM-5 Measures: The clinician thinks about the singular's side effects to the rules illustrated in the Analytic and Factual Manual of Mental Issues, fifth release (DSM-5), which gives the authority of symptomatic models to ADHD.

Length and Impedance: To make a finding, the side effects probably continued for a specific span (regularly something like a half year) and must essentially debilitate everyday working.

Differential Conclusion: The clinician recognizes the three subtypes of ADHD: Prevalently Scatterbrained Show, Dominatingly Hyperactive-Incautious Show, or Joined Show.

Treatment Arranging: Whenever determined to have ADHD, the medical care proficient examines therapy choices, which might incorporate conducting treatment, drugs, or a mix of both.

Recall that an exact ADHD finding requires a prepared medical care supplier, and it's critical to look for proficient assistance if you suspect you or somebody you know might have ADHD.

Chapter 1: Parenting Strategies

Positive Parenting Techniques

Positive nurturing strategies for youngsters with ADHD (Consideration Shortfall/Hyperactivity Issue) can be exceptionally compelling. Here are a few techniques:

Clear Correspondence: Keep up with open, clear, and reliable correspondence with your youngster. Make sense of assumptions and outcomes smoothly.

Routine and Design: Lay out a day-to-day daily practice with set times for feasts, schoolwork, and sleep time. Consistency assists youngsters with ADHD.

Break Undertakings into More Moderate Advances: Assist your youngster with breaking errands into more modest, sensible moves toward forestalling feeling overpowered.

Utilize Visual Guides: Visual timetables, diagrams, and clocks can help your kid understand and oversee time.

Encouraging feedback: Award acceptable conduct with recognition and little impetuses. Uplifting feedback frequently works better compared to discipline.

Undivided attention: Practice undivided attention to figure out your youngster's considerations and sentiments. Urge them to articulate their thoughts.

Limit Interruptions: Establish a climate with negligible interruptions during schoolwork or other-centered exercises.

Show Self-Guideline: Assist your kid with creating self-guideline abilities, similar to profound breathing or enjoying short reprieves when required.

Prescription Administration: Whenever endorsed, guarantee predictable and legitimate drugs to the executives as exhorted by a medical care proficient.

Look for Help: Join support gatherings or look for direction from experts who have practical experience in ADHD to learn more procedures and adapting strategies.

Recall that each kid is special, and it might require investment to track down the best techniques for your youngster with ADHD. Tolerance, sympathy, and a steady climate are critical.

Creating a Supportive Environment

Establishing a strong climate for ADHD includes understanding and obliging the one-of-a-kind requirements of people with ADHD. Here are a few hints:

Training: Find out about ADHD to more readily comprehend the difficulties it presents and its possible assets.

Structure: Layout schedules and timetables to assist with using time effectively and in association.

Clear Correspondence: Utilize clear and succinct guidelines, and keep up with open lines of correspondence.

Break Assignments into More Moderate Advances: Assist people with ADHD with overseeing errands by breaking them into more modest, more reasonable advances.

Limit Interruptions: Make a messiness-free work area and limit interruptions to the help center.

Give Uplifting feedback: Energize and remunerate little accomplishments to support inspiration.

Steady Apparatuses: Consider devices like coordinators, organizers, or applications intended for ADHD executives.

Adaptability: Be versatile and take into account breaks or changes when required.

Medicine and Treatment: Investigate treatment choices like drug and treatment, if proper.

Empower Actual work: Normal activity can assist with overseeing side effects.

Obvious Signs: Utilize visual guides like schedules, agendas, or a variety of coding to improve the association and use time effectively.

Task Prioritization: Assist with focusing on errands by significance and cutoff time to try not to feel overpowered.

Taking care of oneself: Empower great rest, nourishment, and exercise propensities, as these can affect ADHD side effects.

Social Help: Encourage a strong organization of loved ones who comprehend ADHD challenges.

Diminish Pressure: Limit unpleasant circumstances and furnish unwinding methods to adapt to uneasiness.

Persistence and Compassion: Show getting it and tolerance during troublesome minutes or mishaps.

Objective Setting: Assist with defining reachable objectives and celebrate achievements en route.

Tactile Contemplations: Know about tangible awarenesses that a few people with ADHD might have and make changes likewise.

Limit Screen Time: Lay out limits on screen time to forestall overstimulation.

Proficient Assistance: Look for direction from ADHD mentors, specialists, or care groups for extra systems and adapting abilities.

Recall that consistency is critical to progressing support. Fitting your way to deal with the singular's particular requirements and inclinations is significant for establishing a successful and strong climate.

Effective Communication

Compelling correspondence with somebody who has ADHD (Consideration Shortage/Hyperactivity Issue) can be upgraded through these systems:

Be Clear and Brief: Keep your messages forthright, staying away from superfluous subtleties or extended clarifications.

Utilize Visual Guides: Viewable signals and updates can assist with passing on data all the more. Think about utilizing graphs, records, or outlines.

Keep in touch: Support-centered consideration by keeping in touch during discussions.

Undivided attention: Show that you're effectively connected by gesturing, summing up what you've heard, and posing and explaining inquiries.

Break Errands into More modest Advances: While talking about undertakings or directions, break them into more modest, sensible moves toward forestalling overpower.

Give Positive Input: Recognize achievements and endeavors to rouse and support confidence.

Limit Interruptions: Pick tranquil, low-interruption conditions for significant conversations.

Use Clocks and Alerts: Set cautions or clocks to assist with using time effectively and task advances.

Show restraint: Comprehend that consideration and concentration might vary, and take into account breaks when required.

Empower Self-Backing: Train people with ADHD to communicate their requirements and inclinations in correspondence.

Recollect that powerful correspondence with somebody with ADHD frequently requires adaptability and sympathy. Tailor your way to deal with their particular necessities and inclinations.

Setting Clear Expectations

Setting clear assumptions for somebody with ADHD can be useful. Here are a few hints:

Impart Plainly: Utilize clear and brief language to convey assumptions, and guarantee the individual comprehends what is generally anticipated of them.

Focus on Errands: Help them recognize and focus on assignments to try not to feel overpowered. Use records or visual guides if important.

Break Undertakings into More Modest Advances: Separate bigger errands into more modest, reasonable moves to make them less overwhelming.

Put forth Reasonable Objectives: Lay out feasible objectives and cutoff times, considering their abilities and restrictions.

Give Updates: Delicate updates or alerts can assist them with keeping focused and dealing with their time successfully.

Make an Everyday Practice: Predictable schedules can be useful in giving construction and decreasing interruptions.

Offer Help: Be patient and deal with support while required, recognizing their difficulties and triumphs.

Utilize Uplifting feedback: Remunerating achievements and advances can inspire.

Adaptability: Be available to changes on a case-by-case basis, as people with ADHD might have shifting capacities and energy levels.

Recall that every individual with ADHD is one of a kind, so fitting your way to deal with their particular necessities and preferences is significant.

Chapter 2: Behavioral Interventions

Behavior Modification Strategies

Changing outwardly techniques for youngsters with ADHD can be useful. Here are a few viable procedures:

Encouraging feedback: Award appropriate conduct with commendation or little compensation to propel them.

Clear Principles and Assumptions: Lay out clear, reliable standards and ramifications for breaking them.

Design and Schedule: Keep an anticipated day-to-day timetable to assist them with remaining coordinated.

Break Assignments into More modest Advances: Separation undertakings into sensible pieces to forestall overpower.

Utilize Visual Guides: Visual times tables or graphs can help with understanding and following schedules.

Using time effectively: Show time usage abilities and use clocks for errands.

Give Quick Criticism: Address conduct issues speedily, so they figure out the association among activities and results.

Limit Interruptions: Make a tranquil, mess-free climate for contemplating or errands.

Medicine: at times, a prescription might be suggested by a medical services professional.

Parental Help: Look for direction from experts and parent support gatherings to all the more likely comprehend and oversee ADHD.

Recall that every youngster is remarkable, so it's fundamental to tailor these techniques to their particular necessities and talk with a medical care supplier or specialist for customized directions.

Reward Systems

Reward frameworks play a significant part in grasping ADHD (Consideration Deficiency Hyperactivity Problem). In people with ADHD, there is many times dysregulation in the cerebrum's prize hardware, which can add to the side effects of negligence, impulsivity, and hyperactivity. Here are a few central issues:

Dopamine Brokenness: The mind's award framework depends on the synapse dopamine. In ADHD, there might be irregularities in the delivery and gathering of dopamine, influencing the mind's capacity to answer prizes and inspiration.

Postponed Satisfaction: People with ADHD frequently battle with deferred delight, favoring prompt prizes over long-haul ones. This can prompt an indiscreet way of behaving and trouble with undertakings requiring persistence.

Drug: Some ADHD meds, similar to energizers (e.g., methylphenidate, amphetamine), can help by expanding dopamine levels, further developing consideration, and lessening impulsivity. These prescriptions can upgrade the mind's award reaction.

Social Mediations: Conduct treatments, like possibility the of executives, can be successful in molding wanted ways of behaving in people with ADHD. These treatments frequently include giving prompt awards for getting done with jobs or displaying proper ways of behaving.

Uplifting feedback: Utilizing encouraging feedback techniques, similar to acclaim, tokens, or little rewards, can be useful in spurring people with ADHD to remain on track and complete errands.

Construction and Schedule: Laying out organized schedules and steady timetables can give a feeling of consistency and pride for people with ADHD, making it simpler for them to deal with their side effects.

Profound Guideline: Showing close-to-home guideline abilities can likewise be vital since profound dysregulation frequently goes with ADHD. Figuring out how to oversee disappointment and uneasiness can work on generally speaking prosperity.

Individual Changeability: It means a lot to take note that the reaction to compensate frameworks and mediations can differ enormously among people with ADHD. Fitting systems to a singular's particular necessities is fundamental.

Understanding and tending to compensate for framework dysregulation is a significant part of overseeing ADHD, both through medicine and social media. A multidisciplinary approach, including medical care experts, instructors, and families, is in many cases the best method for supporting people with ADHD.

Time-Outs and Consequences

Kids with ADHD (Consideration Shortfall/Hyperactivity Problem) may battle with motivation control, prompting challenges in dealing with their way of behaving. Breaks and results can be successful techniques for dealing with their way of behaving:

Breaks: Breaks include briefly eliminating the kid from a circumstance when they show an unseemly way of behaving. This can allow them an opportunity to quiet down and ponder their activities. Remember these tips:

Keep breaks short and age-proper (commonly 1 moment each extended period old enough).

Utilize an assigned calm space for breaks.

Makes sense why the break is occurring and what conduct needs to change.

Results: Consistency is key while involving ramifications for youngsters with ADHD:

Lay out clear principles and assumptions.

Execute a prize framework for a positive way of behaving, like a symbolic framework or a graph.

Reliably apply outcomes when rules are broken, however, keep them proportionate and useful (e.g., loss of honors).

Look for Proficient Direction: It means a lot to work with medical services experts, similar to pediatricians or youngster therapists, to make a customized plan for overseeing ADHD. They can offer techniques, drugs (if suitable), and support.

Organized Everyday Practice: Laying out a predictable day-to-day schedule can be especially useful for youngsters with ADHD. Unsurprising timetables can diminish impulsivity and give a feeling of dependability.

Encouraging feedback: notwithstanding ramifications for the negative way of behaving, underscore encouraging feedback. Acclaim and award acceptable conduct expeditiously to persuade your youngster to pursue better decisions.

Correspondence: Keep up with open and compassionate correspondence with your youngster. Urge them to communicate their sentiments and dissatisfactions. This can assist you with grasping their viewpoint and tracking down additional compelling arrangements.

Break Assignments into More Modest Advances: Kids with ADHD might battle with errands that require supported consideration. Break undertakings into more modest, sensible advances and give clear directions to assist them with succeeding.

Drug The executives: A few youngsters with ADHD benefit from prescription recommended by a medical services proficient. Drugs can assist with further developing concentration and drive control. Examine this choice with your kid's primary care physician if you haven't as of now.

Parental Help: Dealing with a youngster with ADHD can challenging. Look for help and schooling for yourself, as a parent or guardian. Nurturing classes and care groups can give significant experiences and techniques.

Consistency and Tolerance: Recall that progress might be slow, and mishaps can occur. Consistency in your methodology and tolerance are fundamental. Celebrate little triumphs and continue to pursue long-haul enhancements.

Individualized Approach: Each youngster with ADHD is one of a kind, so tailor your procedures to their particular requirements and qualities. What works for one kid may not work for another.

Proficient Direction: Keep on talking with medical care experts and experts who can offer continuous appraisal and direction. They can change methodologies and intercessions depending on the situation.

In general, overseeing ADHD in kids requires a diverse methodology that joins social systems, support, and sometimes medicine. Working intimately with medical services experts and remaining informed about the most recent explorations and treatments can significantly help your youngster's prosperity.

Managing Impulsivity and Hyperactivity

Directing impulsivity and hyperactivity in ADHD regularly incorporates a blend of frameworks and interventions. The following are a couple of techniques that can be valuable:

Medication: Insight clinical benefits capable of remedy decisions like energizers (e.g., methylphenidate) or non-energizers (e.g., atomoxetine) that can help with managing secondary effects.

Social treatment: Mental direct treatment (CBT) and changing superficial techniques can prepare individuals with ADHD to see and control rash approaches to acting.

Coordinated plans: Spread out consistent regular timetables to give a sensation of consistency and plan, which can help with decreasing impulsivity and hyperactivity.

Time use techniques: Use mechanical assemblies like tickers, cautions, and timetables to break tasks into reasonable pieces and stay on track.

Affiliation capacities: Educate and practice affiliation capacities to reduce disregard and impulsivity, such as using plans and organizing workspaces.

Care and loosening up strategies: Care reflection and loosening up exercises can help individuals with ADHD manage pressure and reduce impulsivity.

Genuine work: Ordinary action can help with positively redirecting hyperactive energy and further foster fixation and balance.

Sponsorship and tutoring: Search for help from guides, support social events, or informational resources for all the more profoundly concentrate on ADHD and reasonable systems.

Diet and sustenance: A couple of individuals track down that dietary changes, such as reducing sugar utilization and extending omega-3 unsaturated fats, can distinctly influence incidental effects.

Rest tidiness: Assurance of good and consistent rest, as the absence of rest can intensify ADHD aftereffects.

Review that the reasonability of these strategies could vary starting with one individual and then onto the next, and it's crucial to work personally with clinical consideration specialists to make a redid arrangement for managing impulsivity and hyperactivity in ADHD.

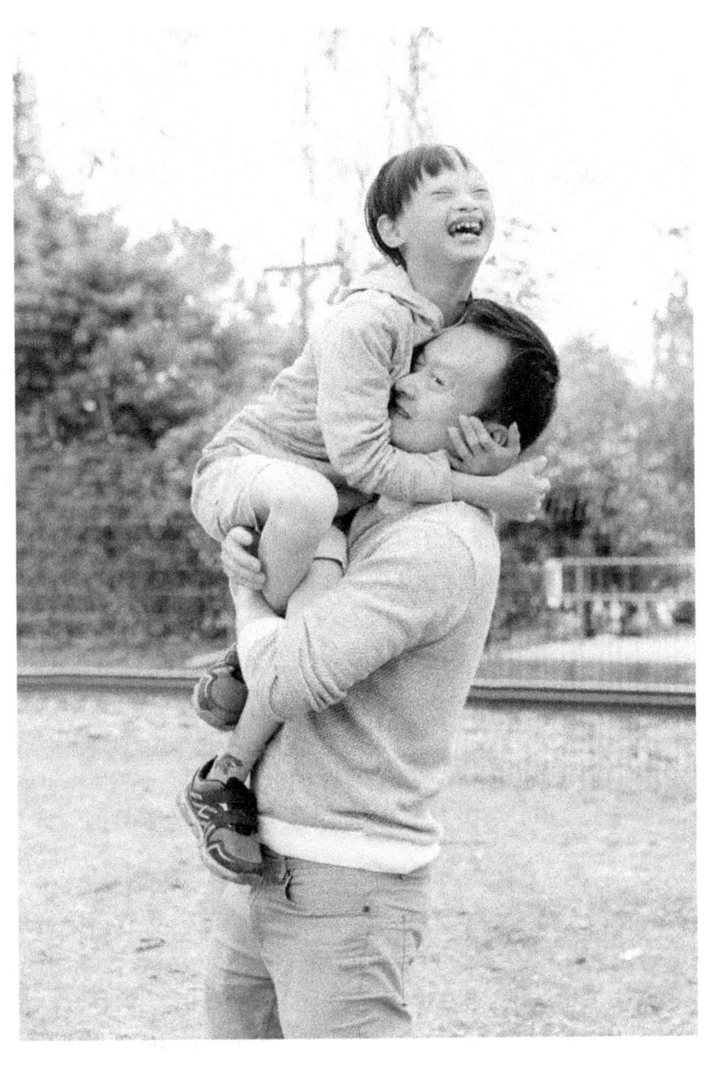

Chapter 3: Medication Options

Medication and ADHD

Prescription is much of the time used to treat ADHD (Consideration Shortfall/Hyperactivity Problem). Normal prescriptions incorporate energizers like methylphenidate (e.g., Ritalin) and amphetamine (e.g., Adderall), as well as non-energizers like atomoxetine (Strattera). Medicine can assist with further developing concentration, consideration, and motivation control in people with ADHD, yet it ought to be recommended and checked by a medical service proficient, as it is viability and secondary effects can differ from one individual to another. Conduct treatment and way of life alterations are likewise significant parts of ADHD treatment.

Energizer Meds: These are the most generally endorsed prescriptions for ADHD. They work by expanding the levels of specific synapses in the mind, which further develops concentration and motivation control. Models incorporate Ritalin, Adderall, and Concerta. They frequently give fast help yet may have potential incidental effects like expanded pulse or sleep deprivation.

Non-Energizer Meds: A few people with ADHD may not answer well to energizers or have specific contraindications. Non-energizer meds like Strattera and guanfacine (Intuniv) are elective choices. They have an alternate component of activity and might be more qualified for specific people.

Individualized Therapy: The decision of prescription ought to be individualized because of an individual's particular necessities, clinical history, and likely secondary effects. A medical services supplier will normally begin with a low portion and change it depending on the situation.

Observing and Secondary effects: Customarily subsequent meet-ups with a medical services supplier are fundamental while taking ADHD drugs. They will screen the prescription's viability and any secondary effects. Incidental effects can differ and may incorporate hunger changes, temperament swings, or expanded pulse.

Long haul Contemplations: ADHD medicine is in many cases some portion of a thorough treatment plan that may likewise incorporate social treatment, guiding, and way of life changes. The objective is to assist people with creating survival techniques and abilities to deal with their side effects.

Security and Abuse: ADHD meds have the potential for abuse, particularly among people without ADHD. Accepting these prescriptions as recommended and not sharing them with others is significant. Abuse can prompt serious well-being chances.

Elective Medicines: Certain individuals investigate elective medicines like dietary changes, neurofeedback, or homegrown supplements. While these methodologies might have a few advantages for specific people, their viability isn't generally settled, and it's urgent to talk with medical services before attempting them.

Kids and Teenagers: ADHD is in many cases analyzed in youth, and the choice to involve prescription in young people ought to include cautious thought and checking by a pediatrician or kid specialist.

Keep in mind, that the decision to involve medicine for ADHD ought to continuously be made in counsel with a certified medical care supplier who can survey what is going on and guide you toward the most suitable therapy plan.

Types of ADHD Medications

There are a few kinds of prescriptions generally used to treat the Consideration Shortage Hyperactivity Issue (ADHD). These can be ordered into:

Energizer Meds:

Methylphenidate-based meds (e.g., Ritalin, Concerta).

Amphetamine-based meds (e.g., Adderall, Vyvanse).

Non-Energizer Meds:

Atomoxetine (Strattera).

Guanfacine (Intuniv).

Clonidine (Kapvay).

The decision of prescription relies upon individual factors and ought to be made in conference with medical care proficient. ADHD prescriptions mean to further develop concentration, consideration, and drive control in people with ADHD.

Methylphenidate-based Drugs:

Ritalin: This short-acting medicine is frequently used to oversee ADHD side effects.

Concerta: It's a lengthy delivery type of methylphenidate, giving longer side effect control.

Amphetamine-based Meds:

Adderall: Joins amphetamine and dextroamphetamine and comes in prompt and expanded discharge structures.

Vyvanse: A prodrug that proselytes to amphetamine in the body and gives a more drawn-out term of activity.

Non-Energizer Prescriptions:

Atomoxetine (Strattera): A particular norepinephrine reuptake inhibitor (NRI) utilized when energizers are inadequate or not liked.

Guanfacine (Intuniv) and Clonidine (Kapvay): Alpha-2 adrenergic agonists that assist with overseeing ADHD side effects by influencing specific receptors in the mind.

Bupropion (Wellbutrin): Albeit essentially a stimulant, bupropion is some of the time utilized off-mark to treat ADHD in grown-ups. It deals with norepinephrine and dopamine synapses.

Dexmethylphenidate (Focalin): Like methylphenidate-based meds, Focalin is an energizer frequently endorsed to oversee ADHD side effects.

Tricyclic Antidepressants: Prescriptions like imipramine and desipramine have been utilized in the past to treat ADHD side effects, however, they are less normally recommended today because of worries about aftereffects.

Conduct Treatment: notwithstanding meds, social treatment, like mental conduct treatment (CBT) or psychoeducation, can be a significant piece of ADHD treatment, particularly in youngsters.

Way of life Changes: Taking on a solid way of life with ordinary activity, a reasonable eating regimen, and satisfactory rest can supplement medicine and treatment in overseeing ADHD side effects.

Recall that the decision of treatment ought to be customized given a singular's particular requirements and inclinations. A conference with a medical care supplier or specialist is critical to deciding the most reasonable therapy plan for ADHD.

Benefits and Risks

ADHD (Consideration Deficiency/Hyperactivity Issue) has two advantages and dangers related with it:

Benefits:

Inventiveness: A few people with ADHD have upgraded their imagination and can consider some fresh possibilities.

Hyperfocus: They can hyperfocus on undertakings they are keen on, prompting expanded efficiency.

Energy: ADHD people frequently have high energy levels, which can be a resource in specific circumstances.

Flexibility: They can be versatile and flourish in powerful conditions.

Excitement: Many are energetic and enthusiastic about their inclinations.

Chances:

Impulsivity: An indiscreet way of behaving can prompt unfortunate independent direction and dangerous activities.

Mindlessness: Trouble centering can influence scholastic and occupation execution.

Close-to-home battles: Emotional episodes and dissatisfaction are normal, influencing connections.

Social difficulties: ADHD might prompt social challenges because of rash or absentminded ways of behaving.

Existing together circumstances: Frequently, ADHD is joined by other emotional well-being issues.

It's vital to take note that the effect of ADHD shifts from one individual to another, and with legitimate help and treatment, people can deal with the dangers and influence the advantages of their interesting qualities.

Benefits:

Innovativeness: ADHD people might have an increased capacity to think imaginatively, making them extraordinary issue solvers and trailblazers.

Hyperfocus: When participate in something they're energetic about, they can hyperfocus for expanded periods, accomplishing great outcomes.

Energy: Their high energy levels can be favorable in actually requesting positions or exercises.

Versatility: ADHD people frequently adjust well to new or changing circumstances because of their adaptability and speedy reasoning.

Energy: They can move toward errands with energy and fervor, which can be infectious and persuade others.

Gambles:

Impulsivity: A rash way of behaving can prompt mishaps, monetary issues, or stressed connections.

Absentmindedness: Trouble supporting consideration can bring about intellectual or expert difficulties, including missed cutoff times and lackluster showing.

Close-to-Home Battles: Emotional episodes, disappointment, and profound dysregulation can influence individual and expert connections.

Social Difficulties: Social associations can be confounded because of imprudent or preoccupied conduct, possibly prompting false impressions and clashes.

Existing together Circumstances: Numerous people with ADHD additionally experience coinciding circumstances like tension, sadness, or substance misuse, which can intensify the difficulties they face.

Successful administration of ADHD frequently includes a mix of procedures, including drug, treatment, and way of life changes. People with ADHD must look for proficient direction and back to assist them with tackling their assets and alleviating the dangers related to the condition.

Working with Healthcare Professionals

Working with medical services experts in ADHD includes coordinated efforts with different specialists to give far-reaching care to people with Consideration Deficiency/Hyperactivity Issues. Here are a few critical parts of this cooperation:

Conclusion and Evaluation: Team up with specialists, therapists, or pediatricians to precisely analyze ADHD through a thorough appraisal, including clinical meetings, side effect assessments, and government-sanctioned tests.

Treatment Arranging: Foster individualized treatment plans, frequently including a blend of conduct mediations, medicine to the executives, and instructive help.

Medicine The board: Work intimately with specialists or pediatricians to screen drug viability, incidental effects, and changes on a case-by-case basis.

Social Treatment: Team up with analysts or conduct specialists to execute conduct mediations, like mental conduct treatment (CBT) or parent preparation, to assist with overseeing ADHD side effects.

Instructive Help: Coordinate with teachers, custom curriculum experts, and school instructors to make facilities and backing plans for understudies with ADHD.

Family Association: Draw in families in the treatment cycle, giving schooling and backing to help them comprehend and oversee ADHD.

Multidisciplinary Group: Frequently, overseeing ADHD requires a group approach, including doctors, advisors, school faculty, and different subject matter experts, contingent upon the singular's necessities.

Continuous Correspondence: Keep up with open correspondence with all elaborate experts to guarantee steady and facilitated care for the person with ADHD.

Remain Informed: Remain refreshed on the most recent exploration and best practices in ADHD the board to give the best consideration.

Recall that coordinated effort and a patient-focused approach are vital to assisting people with ADHD to accomplish their best results.

Chapter 4: School and Education

ADHD in the Classroom

Supporting understudies with ADHD in the homeroom can be fundamental for their prosperity. Methodologies might incorporate clear schedules, limiting interruptions, giving breaks, and offering uplifting feedback. It's additionally vital to speak with guardians and consider individualized schooling plans (IEPs) or 504 designs to address their particular requirements.

Organized Climate: Make an efficient and organized study hall with clear assumptions, plans, and viewable prompts.

Seat Position: Seat the understudy with ADHD close to the front of the class and away from interruptions like windows or entryways.

Breaks: Permit short, successive breaks to assist them with overseeing anxiety and keeping up with the center.

Multisensory Learning: Consolidate different instructing techniques that draw in various faculties, like involved exercises or intuitive examples.

Uplifting feedback: Utilize a prize framework to persuade and support acceptable conduct and accomplishments.

Individualized Guidance: Designer your training techniques to oblige their learning style and speed.

Standard Registrations: Give amazing open doors to the understudy to check in with you secretly to talk about their advancement and concerns.

Cooperation: Work intimately with guardians, custom curriculum experts, and instructors to make a strong group for the understudy.

Prescription Administration: If the understudy is taking a drug, guarantee it's controlled as endorsed and screen its adequacy.

Adaptability: Be adaptable and patient, understanding that their necessities might change from one day to another.

Keep in mind, that each understudy with ADHD is extraordinary, so it's essential to individualize your methodology given their particular difficulties and qualities.

Individualized Education Plans (IEPs)

Individualized Training Plans (IEPs) for understudies with ADHD are customized plans intended to meet their particular instructive requirements. These plans are commonly evolved by a group that incorporates educators, guardians, and different trained professionals. Here are a few critical contemplations for IEPs in ADHD:

Evaluation: The cycle starts with an extensive appraisal of the understudy's assets and difficulties connected with ADHD. This might incorporate contributions from guardians, educators, and instructive analysts.

Clear Objectives: IEPs frame clear, quantifiable objectives custom-fitted to the understudy's novel requirements. These objectives frequently address scholastic, conduct, and social perspectives.

Facilities and Changes: The IEP might incorporate facilities and alterations to help the understudy's learning. Facilities could incorporate broadened time for tasks or tests, particular seating, or admittance to assistive innovation. Adjustments might include modifying the educational program to more readily suit the understudy's requirements.

Conduct Intercessions: Procedures for overseeing ADHD-related ways of behaving are significant. This could include conducting intercessions, self-guideline methods, or interactive abilities preparation.

Correspondence and Cooperation: Viable correspondence among all colleagues is fundamental. Standard gatherings and updates guarantee that the IEP stays pertinent and versatile to the understudy's advancement.

Support Administrations: Understudies with ADHD might profit from extra help administrations, like directing, language training, or word-related treatment, which can be remembered for the IEP.

Progress Observing: IEPs ought to incorporate a framework for following the understudy's advancement toward their objectives, considering changes on a case-by-case basis.

Progress Arranging: For more seasoned understudies, change arranging sets them up for life past a school, including post-auxiliary instruction or business.

Recall that an IEP is a legitimately restricting report, and schools are committed to offering the types of assistance and facilities determined. Guardians and gatekeepers assume a significant part in supporting their youngsters' requirements and guaranteeing that the IEP is successfully executed.

Teacher–Parent Collaboration

Individualized Training Plans (IEPs) for understudies with ADHD are customized plans intended to meet their particular instructive requirements. These plans are commonly evolved by a group that incorporates educators, guardians, and different trained professionals. Here are a few critical contemplations for IEPs in ADHD:

Evaluation: The cycle starts with an extensive appraisal of the understudy's assets and difficulties connected with ADHD. This might incorporate contributions from guardians, educators, and instructive analysts.

Clear Objectives: IEPs frame clear, quantifiable objectives custom-fitted to the understudy's novel requirements. These objectives frequently address scholastic, conduct, and social perspectives.

Facilities and Changes: The IEP might incorporate facilities and alterations to help the understudy's learning. Facilities could incorporate broadened time for tasks or tests, particular seating, or admittance to assistive innovation. Adjustments might include modifying the educational program to more readily suit the understudy's requirements.

Conduct Intercessions: Procedures for overseeing ADHD-related ways of behaving are significant. This could include conducting intercessions, self-guideline methods, or interactive abilities preparation.

Correspondence and Cooperation: Viable correspondence among all colleagues is fundamental. Standard gatherings and updates guarantee that the IEP stays pertinent and versatile to the understudy's advancement.

Support Administrations: Understudies with ADHD might profit from extra help administrations, like directing, language training, or word-related treatment, which can be remembered for the IEP.

Progress Observing: IEPs ought to incorporate a framework for following the understudy's advancement toward their objectives, considering changes on a case-by-case basis.

Progress Arranging: For more seasoned understudies, change arranging sets them up for life past a school, including post-auxiliary instruction or business.

Recall that an IEP is a legitimately restricting report, and schools are committed to offering the types of assistance and facilities determined. Guardians and gatekeepers assume a significant part in supporting their youngsters' requirements and guaranteeing that the IEP is successfully executed.

Study Tips for Children with ADHD

Unquestionably! Here are some review tips that can be useful for youngsters with ADHD:

Make a Predictable Everyday Practice: Lay out a day-to-day plan with an assigned concentration on times. Consistency can assist with further developing concentration and consideration.

Break Undertakings into More Modest Advances: Separation tasks into more modest, sensible errands. This makes it less overpowering and simpler to keep focused.

Utilize Visual Guides: Visual guides like bright outlines, charts, and cheat sheets can make concentrating captivating and assist with maintenance.

Give an Interruption-Free Climate: Limit interruptions by picking a calm, mess-free spot to study. Consider commotion-dropping earphones if necessary.

Use Clocks and Alerts: Set clocks to work so, engaged explodes (e.g., 20-30 minutes) trailed by brief breaks. This can further develop focus.

Integrate Development: Take into account short development breaks during and concentrate on meetings. Actual work can assist youngsters with ADHD to pull together.

Coordinate Materials: Show hierarchical abilities, like utilizing folios, envelopes, and computerized instruments to monitor tasks and due dates.

Execute Encouraging feedback: Offer awards for following through with responsibilities or accomplishing concentrate on objectives to persuade and build up great review propensities.

Think about Medicine and Treatment: Talk with medical services proficient about drug or treatment choices if suitable for your youngster's particular necessities.

Look for Help: Team up with educators, school instructors, and custom curriculum administrations to make an individualized training plan (IEP) if vital.

Put forth Reasonable Objectives: Assist your youngster with defining attainable objectives for each study meeting. Separate bigger objectives into more modest, reasonable errands.

Use Multisensory Learning: Integrate various faculties into learning, for example, paying attention to book recordings, drawing outlines, or utilizing active materials.

Care and Unwinding: Show unwinding procedures like profound breathing or care activities to assist with diminishing nervousness and further develop the center.

Focus on Subjects: Distinguish the most difficult subjects or assignments and tackle them during the times when your youngster's center is at its ideal.

Give Clear Guidelines: Utilize compact and clear directions for tasks and undertakings to forestall disarray.

Empower Self-Observing: Train your youngster to perceive indications of interruption and foster procedures to freely pull together.

Utilize Positive Language: Offer consolation and uplifting feedback instead of analysis while talking about concentrating on propensities.

Make a Schoolwork Agenda: A visual agenda can help your youngster track and complete tasks bit by bit.

Consider Inventive Review Strategies: Let your youngster investigate different review techniques like brain planning, pretending, or making tunes to recall data.

Ordinary Activity and Rest: Guarantee your kid gets customary actual work and adequate rest, as both assume an urgent part in overseeing ADHD side effects.

Limit Screen Time: Decrease screen time and support parts from electronic gadgets to forestall overstimulation.

Think about a Review Mate: Collaborating with a friend for examining can give inspiration and responsibility.

Speak with Educators: Keep open correspondence with instructors to remain informed about your youngster's advancement and any extra help required.

Observe Accomplishments: Celebrate little triumphs and achievements in your kid's review process to support their certainty.

Recollect that what works best might change starting with one youngster and then onto the next, so it's essential to explore different avenues regarding these procedures and adjust them to your kid's particular necessities and inclinations. Consistently reconsider and change the methodology as important to help their learning and prosperity.

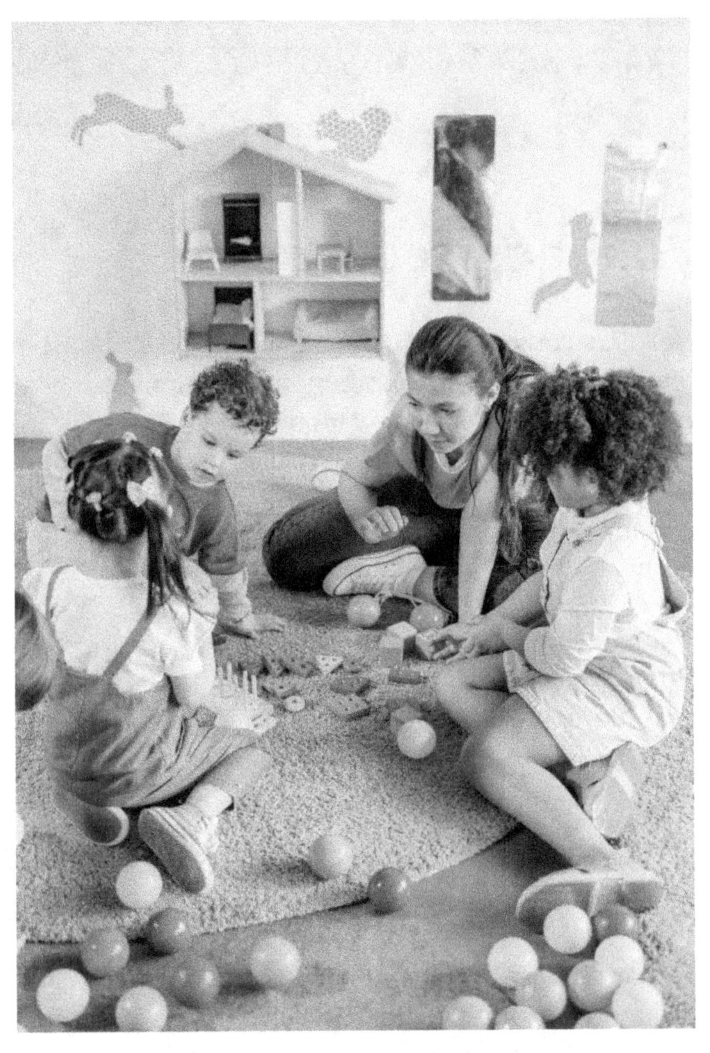

Chapter 5: Emotional and Social Development

Building Self-Esteem

Building confidence in people with ADHD can be testing, however, it's fundamental for their general prosperity. Here are a few techniques:

Recognize Their Assets: Help them perceive and commend their abilities to interest and gifts. Center around their assets instead of harping on shortcomings.

Put forth Practical Objectives: Urge them to lay out feasible objectives, both present moment and long haul. Little triumphs can support confidence.

Offer Help: Offer basic encouragement and consolation. Tell them that you have faith in their capacities.

Foster Survival methods: Work together to foster systems for overseeing ADHD side effects. This can prompt a feeling of control and achievement.

Advance Mindfulness: Assist them with understanding their ADHD and what it means for them. Mindfulness can lessen self-fault and increment self-acknowledgment.

Energize Inspiration: Advance a positive outlook. Instruct them to reexamine negative considerations and spotlight on their achievements.

Interactive abilities Preparing: Work on interactive abilities to encourage positive connections, which can add to confidence.

Look for Proficient Assistance: Consider treatment or guiding, for example, mental conduct treatment, which can address confidence issues connected with ADHD.

Drug and Therapy: Guarantee they are getting suitable clinical treatment for ADHD side effects, which can make confidence-building attempts more viable.

Establish a Steady Climate: Encourage a climate at home and in school or work that is understanding and obliging of their necessities.

Recall that building confidence is a continuous interaction, and advancement might be progressive. Tolerance and reliable help are vital.

Coping with Frustration

Adapting to disappointment in ADHD can be testing, yet some methodologies can help:

Perceive Triggers: Distinguish what circumstances or assignments will quite often disappoint you the most. Understanding your triggers can help you expect and plan for them.

Break Errands into More Modest Advances: Gap enormous undertakings into more modest, more reasonable advances. This can make it simpler to remain on track and lessen dissatisfaction.

Utilize Visual Updates: Utilize visual guides like daily agendas, schedules, and suggestions to assist you with remaining coordinated and on target.

Using time effectively: Set clocks or cautions to designate explicit time spans for errands. This can keep you from becoming overpowered.

Care and Unwinding Strategies: Practice care contemplation or profound breathing activities to quiet your psyche when disappointment fabricates.

Look for Help: Converse with companions, family, or a specialist who can offer close-to-home help and systems for overseeing dissatisfaction.

Medicine: at times, a prescription recommended by medical care proficient can assist with overseeing ADHD side effects, including impulsivity and dissatisfaction.

Practice and Sound Way of Life: Customary active work and a reasonable eating regimen can emphatically influence your mindset and consideration.

Reward Framework: Make a prize framework for following through with jobs or arriving at objectives to give inspiration and a feeling of achievement.

ADHD Instructing: Consider working with an ADHD mentor who can give customized methodologies and direction.

Recall that what turns out best for overseeing disappointment might change from one individual to another, so finding techniques that suit your singular requirements and preferences is fundamental. Talking with a medical care proficient who has some expertise in ADHD can likewise be helpful.

Time-Hindering: Allot explicit blocks of time for various undertakings or exercises. This can assist you with keeping on track and forestall performing various tasks, which can prompt disappointment.

Limit Interruptions: Make a messiness-free and coordinated work area. Using surrounding sound-blocking earphones or background noise important to lessen interruptions.

Use Innovation Carefully: Use applications and devices intended for ADHD, for example, task chiefs or center applications, to assist with association and using time productively.

Practice Persistence: Comprehend that progress might be slower now and again, and enjoying reprieves when disappointment builds is alright. Show restraint toward yourself.

Mindfulness: Focus on your body and psyche. If you feel disappointment rising, pause for a minute to survey your feelings and settle on a strategy.

Social Help: Offer your difficulties and objectives with a believed companion or relative who can offer support and responsibility.

Rest Cleanliness: Guarantee you get sufficient soothing rest as exhaustion can compound ADHD side effects and disappointment.

Journaling: Keep a diary to record your considerations and feelings. This can assist you with acquiring bits of knowledge into examples of dissatisfaction and how to address them.

Careful Development: Take part in exercises like yoga or judo, which join actual development with care to further develop the center and diminish pressure.

Adaptability: Embrace adaptability and versatility in your way of dealing with assignments and objectives. In some cases, it's OK to change plans if it prompts a more useful result.

Recall that overseeing ADHD and dissatisfaction is a continuous cycle, and it's critical to show restraint toward yourself as you try different things with various systems to find what turns out best for you. Talking with a psychological well-being proficient with skill in ADHD can give significant direction and backing custom-made to your particular necessities.

Developing Social Skills

Creating interactive abilities in people with ADHD can be testing however useful. Think about these procedures:

Organized Social Exercises: Participate in organized bunch exercises or clubs to rehearse social connections.

Pretending: Use pretend to mimic social circumstances and practice proper reactions.

Social Training: Look for direction from a specialist or mentor experienced in ADHD and interactive abilities.

Undivided attention: Work on undivided attention abilities to all the more likely grasp others in discussions.

Mindfulness: Empower mindfulness of ADHD side effects and their effect on friendly communications.

Care: Practice care to further develop concentration and motivation control in friendly circumstances.

Medicine and Treatment: Consider drug and treatment as a component of a thorough treatment plan.

Uplifting feedback: Prize yourself or your youngster for fruitful social communications to build up a sure way of behaving.

Social Stories: Utilize social stories to show proper social ways of behaving and reactions.

Persistence: Comprehend that progress might be continuous, and it's vital to be patient and tireless.

Interactive abilities Gatherings: Join or sign up for interactive abilities bunches explicitly intended for individuals with ADHD. These gatherings give a steady climate to rehearse and learn.

Visual Guides: Utilize visual guides, for example, social conduct diagrams or feeling cards, to help perceive and answer expressive gestures.

Separate Errands: Separate complex social connections into more modest, sensible moves toward making them less overpowering.

Practice Sympathy: Work on understanding others' viewpoints and sentiments to fabricate compassion.

Put forth Practical Objectives: Put forth reachable social objectives and track progress to remain inspired.

Using time productively: Further, develop time usage abilities to lessen impulsivity and be more dependable in group environments.

Social Contents: Plan and practice prearranged reactions for normal social circumstances, similar to good tidings or casual conversation.

Peer Backing: Interface with other people who have ADHD to impart encounters and systems for adapting to social difficulties.

Social Applications and Games: Investigate applications and games intended to assist with working on interactive abilities in a tomfoolery and intelligent way.

Family Backing: Include relatives simultaneously, so they can give understanding and backing.

Recollect that creating interactive abilities is a progressive cycle, and celebrating little triumphs en route is fundamental. Tailor these systems to the singular's particular requirements and look for direction from experts who have some expertise in ADHD when vital.

Dealing with Bullying

Managing harassment when you have ADHD can be testing, however, there are methodologies you can utilize:

Look for Help: Converse with a confided-in grown-up, like a parent, educator, or school guide, about the tormenting you're encountering. They can give direction and backing.

Assemble Confidence: Work on building your fearlessness and confidence. This can make you to a lesser extent an objective for menaces and assist you with adapting better to their activities.

Acquire Adapting Abilities: Foster survival methods for managing pressure and tormenting. This could incorporate unwinding methods, care, or taking part in exercises you appreciate.

Instruct Others: Assist with instructing your friends, educators, and school staff about ADHD. Expanding mindfulness can prompt more prominent comprehension and backing.

Emphaticness Preparing: Figure out how to advocate for yourself tranquility and unhesitatingly without being forceful. This can dissuade menace and assist you with defending yourself.

Keep away from Segregation: Make an effort not to detach yourself. Invest energy with companions who support you and offer your inclinations.

Report Episodes: Track harassing occurrences and report them to school specialists. They should address harassment.

Proficient Assistance: If the harassment is causing serious profound trouble, consider looking for help from an emotional well-being proficient person who has practical experience in ADHD or tormenting.

Join Care Groups: Search out help gatherings or online networks for people with ADHD. Interfacing with other people who face comparable difficulties can give solace and guidance.

Compromise Abilities: Acquire compromise abilities to assist you with tending to harassing circumstances calmly. Here and there, self-assured correspondence and critical thinking can determine issues.

Remain Informed: Grasp your privileges and the counter-harassing strategies in your everyday schedule. Information on these arrangements can enable you to make a suitable move.

Practice Care: Care procedures can assist you with remaining grounded and overseeing pressure. It can likewise work on your profound strength even with harassment.

Include Guardians: If you're a parent of a youngster with ADHD who's encountering harassment, team up intimately with the school and educators to guarantee your kid's security.

Support Open Correspondence: Urge your kid to discuss their encounters with ADHD and harassment. A steady and understanding climate at home can have a major effect.

Report Everything: Keep a point-by-point record of harassing occurrences, including dates, times, areas, and witnesses. This documentation can be essential while revealing the torment.

Self-Support Abilities: Show your youngster self-backing abilities, assisting them with communicating their requirements and limits to other people, including instructors and friends.

Think about Treatment: Treatment, like mental conduct treatment (CBT), can assist people with ADHD foster survival methods, and address inner difficulties connected with harassment.

Empower Positive Interests: Urge your kid to seek leisure activities and interests they are enthusiastic about. This can help their confidence and give a departure from tormenting related pressure.

Keep in mind that tending to harass frequently requires a blend of techniques, and it might require investment. Keep the lines of correspondence open with believed people who can uphold you, and make sure to provide proficient assistance if necessary.

Chapter 6: Healthy Lifestyle Habits

Nutrition and Diet

Nourishment and diet can assume a part in overseeing ADHD (Consideration Deficiency Hyperactivity Issue), although they are not a swap for clinical treatment. A few dietary contemplations for ADHD might include:

Omega-3 Unsaturated fats: A few examinations propose that omega-3 unsaturated fats tracked down in fish and flaxseed may decidedly affect ADHD side effects.

Protein: Including lean protein sources like poultry, fish, beans, and tofu in the eating regimen might assist with balancing out glucose levels and further develop the center.

Complex Starches: Food varieties with complex carbs, like entire grains and vegetables, can give a consistent stock of energy and may assist with fixation.

Restricting Sugar and Counterfeit Added Substances: A few people with ADHD might be sensitive to sugar and fake added substances, so decreasing these in the eating routine might be helpful.

Normal Feasts: Eating customary, adjusted dinners and tidbits can assist with keeping up with stable glucose levels and forestall mindset swings.

Hydration: Remaining very hydrated is significant for generally speaking mind capability and fixation.

Micronutrients: Satisfactory admission of fundamental nutrients and minerals is essential. At times, supplementation with supplements like zinc, iron, magnesium, and vitamin D might be suggested, however, this ought to be finished under clinical watch.

Caffeine: While moderate caffeine utilization might further develop the center in certain people, extreme caffeine admission can diminish side effects. Checking caffeine admission, particularly in children is significant.

Food Awarenesses and Sensitivities: Certain individuals with ADHD might have responsive qualities or aversions to specific food sources, like gluten or dairy. Distinguishing and taking out these trigger food sources from the eating regimen might prompt side effect improvement.

Glycemic File: Picking food sources with a lower glycemic record (GI) can assist with settling glucose levels and forestall energy crashes. Low-GI food sources incorporate entire grains, vegetables, and non-dull vegetables.

Feast Timing: Having organized dinner and tidbit times can assist with controlling energy levels and forestall peevishness and impulsivity.

Hydration: Parchedness can influence focus and state of mind. Support normal water admission for the day.

Individual Variety: It's memorable's essential that not all people with ADHD will answer the same way to dietary changes. What works for one individual may not work for another, so a customized approach is critical.

At last, overseeing ADHD through sustenance and diet is a perplexing and individualized process. Talking with medical care proficiently, taking into account a food journal to follow possible triggers, and intently checking the impacts of dietary changes on ADHD side effects can be in every way supportive moves toward tracking down the best dietary methodology.

Exercise and Physical Activity

Practice and active work can emphatically affect people with ADHD (Consideration Deficiency Hyperactivity Issue). Here are a few advantages:

Further developed Concentration: Active work can expand the arrival of synapses like dopamine and norepinephrine, which can upgrade concentration and consideration in people with ADHD.

Decreased Impulsivity: Ordinary activity might assist with diminishing impulsivity and hyperactivity, which are normal side effects of ADHD.

Stress Decrease: Exercise can mitigate pressure and tension, which frequently coincide with ADHD.

Better Rest: Actual work can advance better rest quality, which is critical for overseeing ADHD side effects.

Chief Capability: Exercise might further develop leader capabilities like preparation, association, and working memory, which are in many cases hindered in people with ADHD.

Prescription Improvement: A few investigations propose that exercise can supplement the impacts of ADHD meds, prompting better side effects across the board.

It's critical to take note that while exercise can be gainful, it's anything but a swap for different medicines, for example, drugs or treatment, that might be important for overseeing ADHD. It's fitting for people with ADHD to talk with medical care experts to make an exhaustive therapy plan. Also, the sort and force of activity ought to be customized to individual inclinations and abilities.

Sleep Management

Overseeing rest in ADHD can be testing, however, it's critical for by and large prosperity. Here are a few hints:

Steady Everyday practice: Lay out a normal rest plan, hitting the hay and awakening at similar times every day, even at the end of the week.

Make a Loosening up Sleep Schedule: Wind down before bed with quieting exercises like perusing, delicate extending, or profound breathing activities.

Limit Screen Time: Keep away from screens (telephones, PCs, televisions) an hour before sleep time, as the blue light can upset rest.

Stay away from Energizers: Decrease caffeine and sugar consumption, particularly in the early evening and night.

Agreeable Rest Climate: Guarantee your room is helpful for rest by keeping it dim, cool, and calm.

Drug The executives: Whenever recommended, take ADHD meds before the day to stay away from impedance with rest.

Work-out Consistently: Participate in active work during the day, yet stay away from extreme activity near sleep time.

Mental Conduct Treatment: Think about CBT-I (Mental Social Treatment for A sleeping disorder) with a specialist who spends significant time on rest issues.

Diet and Nourishment: Keep a decent eating regimen and keep away from weighty feasts near sleep time.

Care and Unwinding: Practice unwinding procedures like reflection to quiet the brain before rest.

Keep a Rest Journal: Track your rest designs, taking note of when you hit the sack, awaken, and any rest unsettling influences. This can assist with distinguishing patterns and regions for development.

Oversee Pressure: Stress and nervousness can demolish rest issues. Foster methods for dealing with especially difficult times, for example, journaling, treatment, or yoga to successfully oversee pressure.

Limit Rests: While short rests can be restored, stay away from long or late-evening rests that can slow down evening rest.

Slow Changes: Assuming that you want to change your rest plan, do it progressively by moving sleep time and wake time by 15-30 minutes every day until you arrive at your ideal timetable.

Normal Light Openness: Get openness to regular light during the day, as it manages your body's inner clock and further develops the best quality.

Stay away from Liquor and Smoking: Both liquor and nicotine can disturb rest, so staying away from them, particularly near bedtime is ideal.

Repetitive Sound Machine: Certain individuals with ADHD find background noise-relieving sounds supportive to overwhelm interruptions and establish a more tranquil rest climate.

Prescription Survey: Consistently talk about your meds with your medical care supplier, as specific ADHD drugs might influence rest, and changes may be fundamental.

Remain Steady: Attempt to keep up with your rest standard, even at the end of the week or during excursions, to assist with controlling your body's interior clock.

Look for Proficient Assistance: On the off chance that rest issues continue to happen regardless of attempting these systems, talk with a rest-trained professional or a medical care supplier experienced in treating rest problems.

Recall that overseeing rest in ADHD frequently requires persistence and experimentation to find what turns out best for you. Tailor these tips to your particular necessities and talk with medical care experts for direction.

Mindfulness and Stress Reduction

Care methods can be useful for people with ADHD to lessen pressure and further develop centers. Rehearses like contemplation and profound breathing can advance mindfulness and better close-to-home guidelines. Nonetheless, it's memorable's essential that ADHD is a neurobiological condition, and keeping in mind that care can be an important device, it may not supplant different medicines like prescription or treatment. Talk with a medical care professional for customized direction.

Care Characterized: Care includes giving centered consideration to the current second without judgment. It can assist people with ADHD to become more mindful of their viewpoints, feelings, and real sensations.

Benefits for ADHD: Care practices can work on poise, consideration, and profound guidelines. This can be especially useful for dealing with the impulsivity and distractibility frequently connected with ADHD.

Stress Decrease: Care can lessen pressure by advancing unwinding and diminishing the effect of stressors. Standard practice can prompt a more settled perspective, making it simpler to deal with the everyday difficulties that can be distressing for people with ADHD.

Viable Procedures: Strategies like care contemplation, profound breathing activities, and body examinations are normally utilized. These activities can be adjusted to suit a singular's requirements and inclinations.

Care-Based Mediations: A few treatments, similar to Care Based Pressure Decrease (MBSR) and Care Based Mental Treatment (MBCT), have been adjusted for ADHD. They consolidate care rehearses with mental conduct methodologies to address ADHD side effects and diminish pressure.

Integral Methodology: Care ought to be viewed as a reciprocal technique instead of a sole treatment for ADHD. It can function admirably close to different medicines like prescription, treatment, and way of life alterations.

Consistency Matters: Consistency is key while rehearsing care. Normal meetings, regardless of whether they are short, can prompt more observable advantages over the long run.

Proficient Direction: It's prudent to gain care methods from a certified educator, particularly on the off chance that you're new to the training or have explicit objectives connected with ADHD the executives.

Recollect that ADHD is an intricate condition, and what works best can change from one individual to another. It's fundamental to talk with a medical care proficient who can assist with making a custom-fitted arrangement for overseeing ADHD and stress.

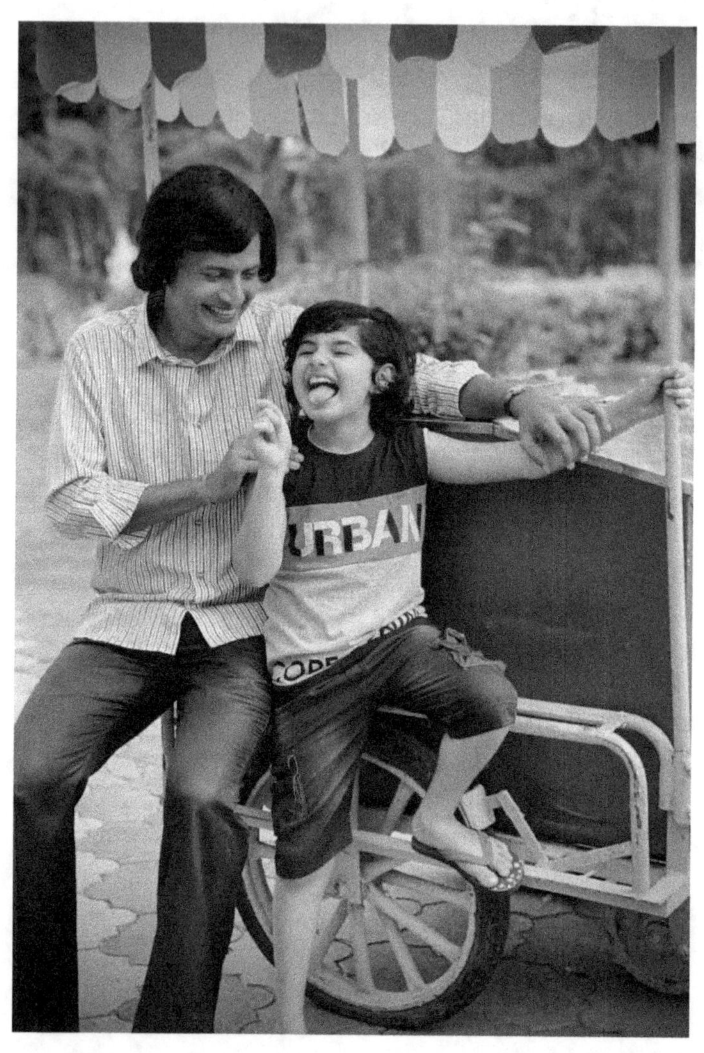URBAN

Chapter 7: Siblings and Family Support

ADHD's Impact on Siblings

ADHD can differentially affect the skin of a kid with ADHD. Here are a few different ways it can influence them:

Consideration Awkwardness: Kin might feel disregarded or dismissed when their folks or parental figures are centered around dealing with the requirements of the youngster with ADHD, which can create sensations of hatred or envy.

Conduct Demonstrating: Kin could impersonate a portion of the ways of behaving or propensities for the youngster with ADHD, both positive and pessimistic, as they notice and collaborate with them consistently.

Expanded Liability: More established kin, specifically, may take on additional obligations, like assisting with schoolwork or offering close-to-home help to their kin with ADHD, which can influence their day-to-day schedules and feelings of anxiety.

Struggle and Dissatisfaction: Kin might encounter clashes with their ADHD kin because of a hasty or problematic way of behaving, prompting stressed connections inside the family.

Understanding and Sympathy: Optimistically, living with kin with ADHD can likewise cultivate more noteworthy figuring out, compassion, and persistence among kin, as they figure out how to adjust to their kin's remarkable requirements.:

Contrasts in Consideration: Kin might see that their folks or parental figures invest more energy in assisting the kid with ADHD with undertakings like schoolwork, treatment meetings, or medical checkups. This inconsistent circulation of consideration can create sensations of injustice.

Scholastic Execution: Kin could feel strain to succeed scholastically to make up for their ADHD kin's difficulties in school. On the other hand, they might battle scholastically because of interruptions or disturbances brought about by their kin.

Social Connections: Kin might confront social difficulties while welcoming companions over or taking part in extracurricular exercises on the off chance that their kin's way of behaving is capricious or troublesome, possibly influencing their public activities.

Close-to-home Effect: Kin might encounter a scope of feelings, including disappointment, shame, or even culpability about feeling adversely towards their ADHD kin. It's significant for guardians to address these feelings and offer close-to-home help.

Support and Instruction: A few kin might become advocates for their ADHD kin, assisting with instructing companions, educators, and others about ADHD to diminish shame and advance comprehension.

Special Bonds: Despite the difficulties, numerous kin of youngsters with ADHD foster exceptional bonds and strength. They might foster a profound feeling of compassion and become more versatile and patient people.

In rundown, ADHD can affect kin, both positive and negative. Open correspondence, basic encouragement, and a steady family climate are fundamental for assisting kin with exploring these difficulties and fabricating solid connections. Furthermore, including kin in the treatment and schooling process about ADHD can encourage understanding and participation inside the family.

Strengthening Family Bonds

Reinforcing family bonds while managing ADHD can be testing yet fundamental. Think about these tips:

Schooling: Find out about ADHD together to all the more likely grasp its belongings and difficulties.

Open Correspondence: Encourage transparent conversations about ADHD-related issues, sentiments, and concerns.

Tolerance: Practice persistence and compassion while managing ADHD-related ways of behaving and difficulties.

Schedule: Lay out reliable schedules and designs to assist with overseeing side effects and diminishing pressure.

Support: Look for help from ADHD subject matter experts, specialists, or care groups to pick up survival methods.

Individualized Approaches: Designer methodologies to every relative's necessities, as ADHD influences everybody unexpectedly.

Uplifting feedback: Perceive and remunerate achievements, regardless of how little, to help confidence.

Quality Time: Hang out doing exercises that advance holding and association.

Taking care of oneself: Guarantee every relative gets some margin for taking care of oneself to diminish pressure and keep up with prosperity.

Adaptability: Be versatile and able to change procedures depending on the situation to accommodate evolving conditions.

Strengthening: Empower relatives with ADHD to take responsibility for treatment and self-administration.

Care: Practice care and stress-decrease strategies as a family to work on profound guidelines.

Objective Setting: Put forth feasible objectives together and celebrate progress collectively.

Limit Screen Time: Screen and cutoff screen time for everybody in the family to advance solid propensities.

Kin Backing: Show kin ADHD and energize sympathy and backing for their impacted relative.

Medicine The board: On the off chance that a drug is essential for the treatment plan, guarantee it's taken as endorsed and screen its belongings.

Reliable Standards: Lay out steady principles and results to give structure and decrease disarray.

Job Displaying: Be a positive good example by exhibiting tolerance, association, and restraint.

Quality Rest: Focus on sound rest propensities for all relatives, as the absence of rest can fuel ADHD side effects.

Observe Contrasts: Embrace the extraordinary qualities and gifts that people with ADHD bring to relational intricacy.

Recollect that ADHD can introduce difficulties, however, it additionally accompanies numerous qualities. By cooperating and offering support, you can reinforce your family bonds and assist every part with flourishing.

Support Groups and Resources

Absolutely! Support gatherings and assets for ADHD (Consideration Shortfall/Hyperactivity Problem) can be exceptionally useful. Here are a few choices:

CHADD (Kids and Grown-ups with Consideration Shortfall/Hyperactivity Problem): CHADD is a notable association that gives data, backing, and promotion to people with ADHD. They have neighborhood parts and online assets.

ADDitude Magazine: This web-based magazine offers articles, online courses, and a local area discussion for people and families impacted by ADHD.

Public Organization of Emotional Well-being (NIMH): NIMH offers far-reaching data about ADHD, research updates, and treatment choices.

Online Gatherings and Facebook Gatherings: There are various internet-based networks and Facebook bunches where people with ADHD and their families share encounters, counsel, and backing.

Treatment and Guiding: Consider working with a specialist or guide who spends significant time on ADHD. They can give procedures and backing customized to your requirements.

Medicine The board: If the drug is important for your treatment plan, talk with an in specialist ADHD to track down the right prescription and measurements for you.

Training Administrations: ADHD mentors can give customized methodologies and back to assist you with overseeing day-to-day existence and accomplishing your objectives.

Books and Digital recordings: There are many books and webcasts on ADHD that offer bits of knowledge and useful hints. A few well-known ones incorporate "Headed to Interruption" by Dr. Edward Hallowell and "The ADHD Digital Broadcast."

Work environment Facilities: If you're in the labor force, consider talking about facilities with your boss, like adaptable booking or work area changes.

Nurturing Backing: Guardians of kids with ADHD can profit from parent-preparing projects and care groups like Parent-to-Parent.

Recall that ADHD is an exceptionally individualized condition, and what turns out best for one individual may not work for another. It's critical to investigate various assets and methodologies to find what suits your particular necessities and conditions. Furthermore, talking with a medical services proficient for customized therapy

Chapter 8: Looking Toward the Future

Adolescence and ADHD

Puberty can be a difficult time for people with ADHD (Consideration Shortage/Hyperactivity Problem). ADHD is a neurodevelopmental problem that influences consideration, drive control, and hyperactivity. During pre-adulthood, the side effects of ADHD can turn out to be more articulated because of hormonal changes and expanded scholarly and social requests. Youths with ADHD must get fitting help, which might incorporate treatment, drugs, and methodologies to work on authoritative abilities and using time productively. Early intercession and a steady climate can incredibly help teenagers with ADHD as they explore this momentary period.

Transitioning to Independence

Changing to freedom can be trying for people with ADHD, however, with the right systems and backing, it's feasible. Here are a few hints:

Put forth Clear Objectives: Characterize your present moment and long-haul objectives. Separate them into more modest, reasonable assignments to try not to feel overpowered.

Make Schedules: Lay out everyday schedules and stick to them. Consistency can assist with using time productively and association.

Use Instruments and Innovation: Use ADHD-accommodating applications and apparatuses for tasks on the board, updates, and schedules to remain coordinated.

Using time productively: Learn time usage strategies, like the Pomodoro Strategy, to increment efficiency and lessen delaying.

Look for Drug or Treatment: Counsel medical services proficient about prescription or treatment choices that can assist with overseeing ADHD side effects and further develop the center.

Mindfulness: Comprehend your assets and shortcomings connected with ADHD. Expand on your assets and track down techniques to work around difficulties.

Remain Coordinated: Use frameworks like a variety of coded envelopes, names, or computerized note-taking applications to monitor significant data and assignments.

Solid Way of Life: Focus on a reasonable eating regimen, normal activity, and satisfactory rest to assist with overseeing ADHD side effects.

Encouraging a group of people: Look for help from companions, family, or care groups who figure out ADHD and can give support and responsibility.

Self-Promotion: Figure out how to advocate for yourself by conveying your necessities to teachers, bosses, or other people who can give fundamental facilities or backing.

Break Errands Into Steps: When confronted with an enormous undertaking, break it into more modest, more sensible advances. This makes it more straightforward to remain focused and try not to feel overpowered.

Utilize Visual Guides: Viewable signs like daily agendas, outlines, and charts can assist you with remaining coordinated and recollecting significant data.

Limit Interruptions: Establish an interruption-free climate while working or examining. Use surrounding sound-blocking earphones or applications that block diverting sites.

Practice Care: Care procedures, like contemplation and profound breathing, can assist with further developing concentration and lessen uneasiness related to ADHD.

Time Obstructing: Allot explicit blocks of time for various assignments or exercises. This can assist you with dispensing your time and staying away from overcommitting.

Gain from Difficulties: Cheer up by misfortunes or slip-ups. All things being equal, view them as any open doors to learn and work on your techniques.

Fabricate Interactive abilities: Work on working on interactive abilities and connections, as solid relational associations can offer significant help and systems administration amazing open doors.

Monetary Administration: Acquire planning and monetary administration abilities to guarantee your monetary autonomy and security.

Profession Arranging: Investigate vocations that line up with your inclinations and assets. Look for vocation advising or mentorship to assist you with settling on informed choices.

Proceeded with Instruction: Consider promoting your schooling or expertise improvement. Deep-rooted learning can open up new doors for individual and expert development.

Remain Informed: Keep awake date on the most recent exploration and techniques for overseeing ADHD. Information can engage you to make informed decisions.

Observe Accomplishments: Recognize and praise your accomplishments, regardless of how little they might appear. Encouraging feedback can help inspire.

Proficient Assistance: If you're battling essentially with ADHD side effects, consider counseling a specialist, specialist, or ADHD mentor for customized direction and backing.

Recall that overseeing ADHD and accomplishing freedom is a progressive interaction. It's OK to look for help and adjust your procedures as you come. What turns out best for one individual with ADHD might not be the same as what works for another, so be patient and adaptable in your methodology.

Preparing for Adult Life

Planning for a grown-up existence with ADHD includes creating methodologies to oversee side effects and prevail in different parts of life. Here are a few hints:

Drug The board: Whenever endorsed, accept ADHD prescription as coordinated to assist with further developing concentration and drive control.

Using time productively: Use devices like schedules, organizers, and applications to arrange errands and cutoff times.

Make Schedules: Lay out everyday schedules to keep up with consistency and construction in your life.

Put forth Practical Objectives: Break assignments into more modest, reasonable advances and put forth feasible objectives.

Look for Help: Interface with a specialist or care groups to pick up survival techniques and gain everyday reassurance.

Focus on Taking care of oneself: Get sufficient rest, eat a reasonable eating regimen, work out consistently, and oversee pressure.

Foster Review Methodologies: Use procedures like time impeding, dynamic perusing, and breaking concentrate on meetings into more limited fragments.

Vocation Arranging: Investigate professions that line up with your assets and interests, and consider uncovering ADHD to businesses if important.

Monetary Administration: Make a spending plan, robotize bill installments, and think about looking for monetary guidance if necessary.

Interactive abilities: Work on correspondence and relational abilities to assemble solid connections.

Recollect that overseeing ADHD is a continuous interaction, and it's fundamental to adjust methodologies to accommodate your extraordinary requirements and conditions. Counseling medical care proficiently can give customized direction.

Success Stories and Inspirations

Unquestionably! ADHD, or Consideration Deficiency Hyperactivity Problem, can introduce difficulties, however, numerous people have made amazing progress and act as motivations. The following are a couple of examples of overcoming adversity:

Michael Phelps: The Olympic swimmer has transparently talked about his ADHD finding. Despite confronting difficulties, he became perhaps one of the most embellished competitors ever.

Richard Branson: The tycoon business visionary behind Virgin Gathering has ADHD. His imaginative reasoning and hazard-taking have prompted various fruitful endeavors.

Simone Biles: The aerobatic genius has ADHD and has won different Olympic gold awards. Her commitment to her game is a motivation to many.

Will. i.am: The performer and maker from The Dark Looked at Peas has ADHD. He's known for his inventiveness and energy for music.

Sir Richard Taylor: Prime supporter of Weta Studio, known for its work on "Ruler of the Rings" and "Symbol," has ADHD. His imagination fundamentally affects the entertainment world.

Jessica McCabe: She runs the YouTube channel "How to ADHD" and offers her encounters and ways to oversee ADHD. Her channel has instructed and moved a large number.

These people exhibit that ADHD doesn't need to be a hindrance to progress. With the right procedures, backing, and assurance, individuals with ADHD can succeed in different fields and make huge commitments to society.

Justin Timberlake: The artist, entertainer, and previous NSYNC part has ADHD. His ability and outcome in media outlets are notable.

Ty Pennington: The television host, craftsman, and originator of shows like "Outrageous Makeover: Home Release" has ADHD. His energy for home improvement and configuration radiates through his work.

Solange Knowles: The artist, lyricist, and entertainer, who is likewise Beyoncé's sister, has

ADHD. She's known for her remarkable melodic style and imagination.

Sir Winston Churchill: The previous State leader of the Unified Realm is accepted to have had ADHD. He drove his country during The Second Great War and is famous for his authority.

Zoe Kravitz: The entertainer, vocalist, and model has ADHD. She has shown up in unmistakable movies like "Distraught Max: Rage Street" and "Phenomenal Monsters: The Wrongdoings of Grindelwald."

Adam Levine: The lead vocalist of Maroon 5 and an adjudicator on "The Voice" has ADHD. His melodic ability and effective professionalism are motivational.

David Neeleman: The business person and organizer behind a few carriers, including JetBlue and Azul Brazilian Aircrafts, has ADHD. He's known for his creative way of dealing with the carrier business.

These people show the way that ADHD can coincide with exceptional accomplishments across different fields. Their accounts act as inspiration for those with ADHD to seek after their interests and objectives sincerely and with versatility.

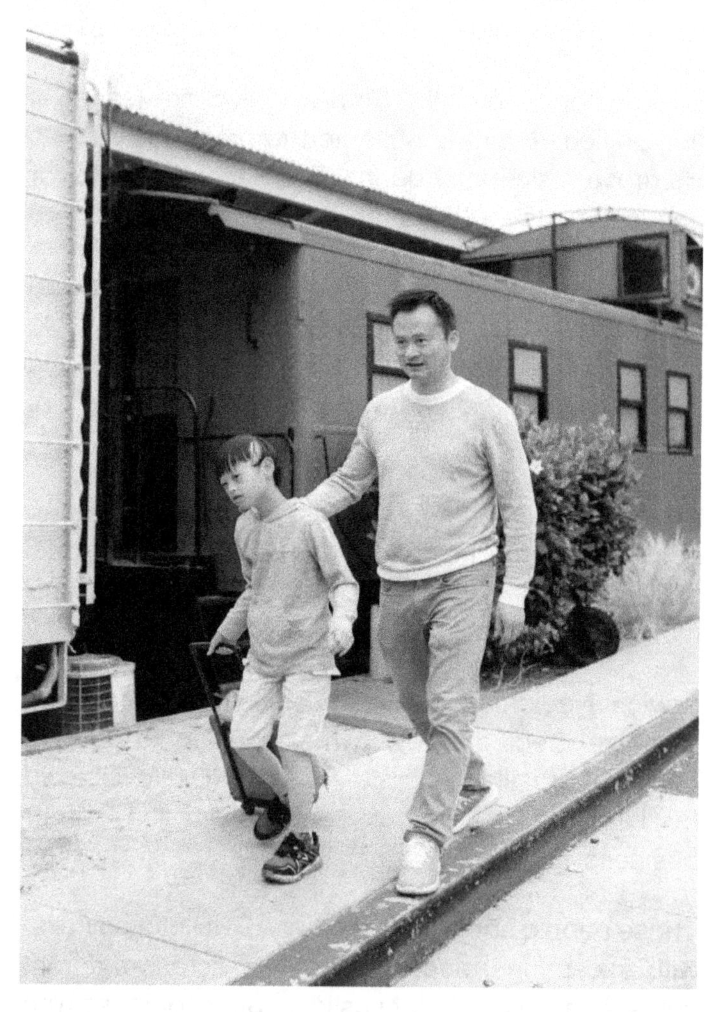

Chapter 9: Comorbid Conditions

Understanding Comorbid Conditions

Comorbid conditions allude to extra clinical or mental problems that coincide with an essential condition, like ADHD (Consideration Shortfall/Hyperactivity Issue). Some normal comorbid conditions in people with ADHD include:

Nervousness Problems: Uneasiness issues like Tension Confusion (Stray), Social uneasiness Issues, or Frenzy Problems oftentimes happen close to ADHD.

Misery: People with ADHD may likewise encounter wretchedness, which can be connected with the difficulties and dissatisfactions related to dealing with their side effects.

Learning Inabilities: Learning problems like dyslexia or dyscalculia frequently co-happen with ADHD and can entangle scholastic execution.

Oppositional Rebellious Turmoil (ODD) and Direct Confusion: These problematic conduct issues can be more normal in kids with ADHD.

Substance Use Problems: Teenagers and grown-ups with ADHD are at higher gamble for substance misuse and habit.

Rest Issues: Rest issues, including sleep deprivation or rest apnea, are normal among those with ADHD.

Tourette Disorder: There is a higher probability of Tourette condition in people with ADHD.

Bipolar Turmoil: Albeit more uncommon, a few people with ADHD may likewise have bipolar confusion.

It's essential to perceive and address comorbid conditions, as they can muddle the administration of ADHD. An extensive evaluation by a medical care proficient is pivotal to give proper therapy and backing customized to a singular's interesting requirements. Treatment frequently includes a blend of social treatment, drug, and backing systems.

Addressing Anxiety and Depression

Tending to tension and wretchedness in people with ADHD regularly includes a multi-layered approach:

Counsel an Expert: Look for help from emotional well-being proficient who has practical experience in ADHD and co-happening conditions. They can give a far-reaching evaluation and treatment plan.

Medicine: Drugs like energizers or non-energizers might assist with overseeing ADHD side effects, which can by implication reduce tension and wretchedness.

Treatment: Mental social treatment (CBT) can be compelling in treating tension and misery. It helps people perceive and change pessimistic idea designs.

ADHD-explicit Systems: Learn methodologies for overseeing ADHD side effects, like using time productively, association, and arranging. This can diminish pressure and work on confidence.

Way of life Changes: A solid way of life with ordinary activity, a fair eating routine, and adequate rest can emphatically influence temperament and in general prosperity.

Support Gatherings: Joining support gatherings or finding a local area for people with ADHD can offer profound help and reasonable exhortation.

Care and Unwinding Strategies: Practices like care contemplation or yoga can assist with overseeing nervousness and work on close-to-home guidelines.

Prescription for Tension/Sadness: at times, medicine explicitly for nervousness or despondency might be fundamental notwithstanding ADHD treatment.

Instructive Help: On the off chance that ADHD influences scholarly or work execution, look for instructive facilities or work environment support.

Customary Development: Keep in touch with your medical care supplier to survey progress and change therapy on a case-by-case basis.

Distinguish Triggers: Comprehend what circumstances or stressors will more often than not deteriorate your nervousness or despondency. Mindfulness can assist you with creating survival methods.

Chief Capability Preparing: Further develop leader capability abilities, which are in many cases weakened in ADHD. This can upgrade your capacity to design, put forth objectives, and oversee everyday undertakings.

Social Help: Fabricate major areas of strength for an organization with loved ones who can offer close-to-home help and support.

Taking care of oneself: Practice taking care of oneself routinely. Participate in exercises you appreciate and that assist you with unwinding, whether it's leisure activities, workmanship, music, or investing energy in nature.

Limit Screen Time: Extreme screen time, particularly via virtual entertainment, can worsen nervousness and wretchedness. Put down certain boundaries and enjoy reprieves.

Journaling: Keeping a diary can assist you with offering your viewpoints and feelings, tracking designs, and distinguishing areas of progress.

A balance between serious and fun activities: Take a stab at a sound balance between serious and fun activities. Overburdening yourself with obligations can add to pressure and state of mind issues.

Careful Acknowledgment: Practice acknowledgment of your ADHD and the difficulties it brings. Self-sympathy and acknowledgment can decrease self-analysis.

Family Training: Teach relatives about ADHD, nervousness, and despondency so they can all the more likely comprehend and uphold you.

Screen Progress: Monitor your advancement and difficulties. Celebrate little triumphs and show restraint toward yourself on troublesome days.

Recollect that overseeing ADHD, nervousness, and despondency is a continuous interaction. It's alright to look for proficient assistance at whatever point required and go ahead and out to your medical care supplier assuming you experience changes in your side effects or general prosperity. Every individual's process is special, and the objective is to find procedures that turn out best for you.

Managing Learning Disabilities

Overseeing learning handicaps in people with ADHD can be testing, however, it's fundamental for their scholarly and self-improvement. Here are a few systems to consider:

Evaluation: Start by getting an exhaustive appraisal to recognize explicit learning incapacities. This might include testing for dyslexia, dyscalculia, or other learning issues.

Individualized Schooling Plan (IEP) or 504 Arrangement: Work with instructors and experts to make a customized plan that tends to the remarkable requirements of the person. These plans might incorporate facilities, adjustments, and objectives to help their learning.

Prescription Administration: For people with both ADHD and learning handicaps, medicine might assist with overseeing ADHD side effects, permitting better concentration and consideration in the homeroom.

Organized Climate: Establish an organized and coordinated learning climate at home and school to lessen interruptions and advance better fixation.

Multisensory Learning: Consolidate multisensory instructing procedures that draw in various faculties (visual, hearable, sensation) to upgrade learning and memory.

Particular Guidance: Search out specific guidance or coaching for the particular learning handicap, like perusing medications for dyslexia.

Innovation Instruments: Use assistive innovation like text-to-discourse programming, discourse-to-message applications, or realistic coordinators to help with perusing, composing, and association.

Consistent encouragement: Offer daily reassurance to address expected disappointment or low confidence related to learning handicaps. Energize a development mentality and flexibility.

Customary Correspondence: Keep up with open correspondence between guardians, educators, and experts to screen headway and make essential acclimations to the instructive arrangement.

Self-Support: Help people with ADHD and learning handicaps to advocate for themselves, figure out their assets and shortcomings, and foster systems to defeat difficulties.

Recall that each individual is interesting, so it's significant to fit the administration's way of dealing with their particular necessities and qualities. A coordinated effort among guardians, teachers, and experts is vital to the outcome of overseeing learning handicaps in ADHD.

Autism Spectrum Disorders and ADHD

Mental imbalance Range Issues (ASD) and Consideration Deficiency Hyperactivity Problem (ADHD) are two unmistakable neurodevelopmental conditions, yet they can now and again co-happen or share specific side effects, prompting covering attributes. The two circumstances are described by difficulties in friendly collaboration and correspondence, however, they contrast in key ways:

Center Highlights:

ASD: Center highlights of ASD remember troubles with social correspondence and association, redundant ways of behaving, limited interests, and tactile responsive qualities.

ADHD: Center elements of ADHD include mindlessness, hyperactivity, and impulsivity.

Social and Correspondence Difficulties:

ASD: People with ASD might have huge difficulties in understanding and exploring social circumstances, frequently battling with nonverbal correspondence and shaping connections.

ADHD: While people with ADHD may likewise experience issues with social collaboration, their essential difficulties are connected with the consideration guidelines and motivation control.

Redundant Ways of behaving:

ASD: Redundant ways of behaving and a solid adherence to schedules or customs are normal in ASD.

ADHD: Redundant ways of behaving are less trait of ADHD; all things considered, impulsivity and hyperactivity are more unmistakable.

Tangible Responsive qualities:

ASD: Numerous people with ASD experience tangible awareness, like uplifted or reduced reactions to tactile improvements (e.g., light, sound, surface).

ADHD: Tactile responsive qualities are not a characterizing component of ADHD.

Beginning and Finding:

ASD: Side effects commonly become obvious from the get-go in adolescence, frequently before age 3. The determination depends on a thorough assessment of conduct and formative history.

ADHD: Side effects of ADHD might be perceived in youth, however, a proper determination is ordinarily made around young. The conclusion depends on unambiguous rules connected with consideration and hyperactivity/impulsivity.

It's critical to take note that while these circumstances have unmistakable attributes, there can be comorbidity, where an individual has both ASD and ADHD. Exact determination and fitted mediations are vital to address the exceptional necessities of people with these circumstances. Assuming that you have explicit inquiries or need more data, kindly go ahead and inquire.

Chemical Imbalance Range Issues (ASD):

Range Nature: ASD is frequently alluded to as a "range" since it envelops a great many side effects seriousness and working levels. A few people with ASD might have huge weaknesses in day-to-day existence, while others might have milder difficulties.

Correspondence Difficulties: Correspondence hardships in ASD can change generally, from nonverbal people to those with cutting-edge language abilities who battle with the nuances of discussion, like figuring out mockery.

Limited Interests: Individuals with ASD frequently foster extreme, explicit interests and may participate in tedious exercises connected with those interests. This is once in a while alluded to as "perseveration."

Early Intercession: Early finding and mediation are urgent for youngsters with ASD. Applied Conduct Investigation (ABA), language instruction, word-related treatment, and interactive abilities preparation are a portion of the medications that can be helpful.

Consideration Shortfall Hyperactivity Problem (ADHD):

Kinds of ADHD: ADHD is arranged into three subtypes: fundamentally distracted show, basically hyperactive-indiscreet show, and joined show

(which incorporates side effects of both heedlessness and hyperactivity-impulsivity).

Leader Working: ADHD is frequently connected with chief capability shortages, which can influence a singular's capacity to design, sort out, oversee time, and complete assignments.

Drug and Social Mediations: Treatment for ADHD might include prescriptions (e.g., energizers like methylphenidate or non-energizers) and conduct intercessions. Prescription can assist with further developing concentration and motivation control, while conduct systems show people adapting abilities.

Life expectancy Effect: ADHD isn't restricted to adolescence; it can persevere into adulthood.

Grown-ups with ADHD might confront difficulties in training, work, and connections on the off chance that their side effects are not overseen.

Existing together Circumstances: ADHD frequently co-happens with different circumstances, like uneasiness, gloom, and learning incapacities. Tending to these comorbidities is fundamental for thorough treatment.

Both ASD and ADHD are perplexing circumstances that can fundamentally influence a singular's life. Early determination and fitting mediations, customized to every individual's exceptional necessities, can have a significant effect on their general prosperity and personal satisfaction. Assuming you have more unambiguous inquiries or need further subtleties, if it's not too much trouble, go ahead and inquire.

Chapter 10: Special Considerations

ADHD in Girls

ADHD (Consideration shortfall/hyperactivity jumble) can frequently show distinctively in young ladies contrasted with young men. Young ladies with ADHD might display side effects like absentmindedness, fantasizing, neglect, and profound excessive touchiness instead of just hyperactivity. This can once in a while prompt underdiagnosis or misdiagnosis. Early acknowledgment and suitable help are vital for overseeing ADHD in young ladies. Assuming that you have explicit inquiries or need more data, go ahead and inquire.

Side effects:

Distractedness: Young ladies with ADHD might battle with concentration, association, and finishing responsibilities. They could frequently commit imprudent errors and experience issues focusing on subtleties.

Hyperactivity-Impulsivity: While hyperactivity is more uncommon in young ladies with ADHD, they can in any case show fretfulness and impulsivity. This could appear as interfering with others, anxiety, or trouble standing by.

Close-to-home Dysregulation: Young ladies with ADHD might encounter serious feelings and emotional episodes. They may be handily disappointed, touchy, or restless. Some likewise display low confidence.

Stalling: Trouble starting undertakings or dawdling is normal. They could battle with using time productively and cutoff times.

The board Systems:

Finding: Early and exact analysis is fundamental. Look for assessment from a medical care proficient who works in ADHD.

Drug: now and again, prescription (e.g., energizers or non-energizers) can assist with overseeing side effects. Talk with a medical care supplier to decide whether it's fitting.

Conduct Treatment: Conduct mediations, like mental social treatment (CBT) or interactive abilities preparation, can be compelling in working on discretion and profound guidelines.

Parental and Educator Backing: Team up with instructors and guardians to think up steady schedules and methodologies for overseeing side effects at home and in school.

Design and Association: Carry out timetables, updates, and visual guides to assist with using time effectively and task consummation.

Daily reassurance: Energize open correspondence about sentiments and give a strong climate to close-to-home articulation.

Solid Way of Life: Advance ordinary activity, a decent eating routine, and adequate rest, as these can assist with mitigating some ADHD side effects.

Instructive Facilities: Investigate Individualized Training Plans (IEPs) or 504 Designs to give scholastic facilities back in school.

Parent Preparing: Consider programs that show guardians successful systems for overseeing ADHD-related ways of behaving.

Recollect that every person with ADHD is novel, and what works best might shift. A custom-fitted methodology with input from medical services experts, teachers, and the actual singular is critical to effective administration.

Cultural and Ethnic Perspectives

Social and ethnic points of view can essentially affect how consideration deficiency hyperactivity jumble (ADHD) is perceived, analyzed, and treated. Here are a few central issues to consider:

Social Variety in Side Effects: The statement of ADHD side effects might fluctuate across societies. For instance, in certain societies, hyperactivity might be less acknowledged and in this way less unmistakable, while negligence or impulsivity might be more recognizable.

Finding and Shame: Various societies might have fluctuating degrees of mindfulness and comprehension of ADHD. In certain societies, there may be shame related to psychological wellness conditions, prompting underdiagnosis or misdiagnosis.

Treatment Approaches: Social convictions and values can impact treatment inclinations. A few families might favor non-pharmacological intercessions, for example, conducting treatment, or over-prescription because of social convictions.

Language Obstructions: Language can be a hindrance to determination and treatment. In multicultural social orders, medical services experts ought to be delicate to language needs and give admittance to mediators if important.

Admittance to Mind: Financial variables and medical care aberrations can influence admittance to ADHD determination and therapy. This can excessively affect minority and low-pay populaces.

Social Ability: Medical care suppliers should be socially skillful, grasping the extraordinary requirements and viewpoints of patients from various social foundations. This incorporates thinking about social convictions regarding emotional well-being and treatment.

Nurturing Styles: Social standards in regards to nurturing styles can impact how ADHD ways of behaving are seen. For instance, a few societies might have stricter discipline, which could influence side effect seriousness.

Local Area Backing: Social and ethnic networks frequently offer help to organizations. Utilizing these organizations can be fundamental in bringing issues to light and working with admittance to focus on people with ADHD.

Research Holes: There might be restricted examination of ADHD in specific social or ethnic gatherings, prompting an absence of comprehension of how the issue appears in those populations.

It's essential to move toward ADHD analysis and treatment with social responsiveness and attention to give even-handed consideration to people from assorted foundations. Fitting meditations to meet the particular necessities and convictions of each social gathering can prompt more viable results.

Giftedness and ADHD

Talent and ADHD (Consideration Shortfall/Hyperactivity Issue) can exist together, yet they are particular circumstances. A few talented people may likewise have ADHD, which can introduce interesting difficulties. It's critical to comprehend and address the two angles to successfully uphold their turn of events. On the off chance that you have explicit inquiries or need more data, kindly go ahead and inquire.

Cross-over: While talent and ADHD are isolated circumstances, there can be a cross-over in qualities. Both can include elevated responsiveness, impulsivity, and extreme concentration, which can make it trying to recognize the two.

Misdiagnosis: Gifted youngsters with ADHD might be misdiagnosed because their qualities can mirror ADHD side effects. Experts must consider the two prospects while assessing a kid's way of behaving and execution.

Exceptional Difficulties: Gifted kids with ADHD might confront extraordinary difficulties. Their extreme spotlight on unambiguous interests can be confused with hyperactivity, and their trouble with errands they find dull might be viewed as obliviousness.

Treatment: Treatment for ADHD in gifted people might require a custom-fitted methodology. Conventional medicine and social mediations might be changed following the youngster's high mental capacities and individual necessities.

Support: Gifted kids with ADHD might profit from a strong and understanding climate that perceives their assets and difficulties. This incorporates proper instructive facilities and techniques to assist them with flourishing scholastically and socially.

Recall that every individual is one of a kind, and an exhaustive evaluation by a medical care proficient or clinician is vital to deciding the most fitting intercessions and backing for a youngster with both skill and ADHD.

ADHD and Trauma

ADHD (Consideration Shortage/Hyperactivity Issue) and injury can now and then be interconnected. Horrendous encounters, particularly during adolescence, may imitate or fuel the side effects of ADHD. Recognizing the two and looking for proficient assistance for a precise finding and suitable treatment is significant. Treatment, drugs, or a blend of both might be suggested relying upon the singular's necessities. On the off chance that you or somebody you know is encountering these issues, counseling emotional well-being proficiently is fundamental for legitimate evaluation and backing.

Side effect Crossover: ADHD and injury can have covering side effects, like challenges with fixation, impulsivity, and profound dysregulation. This crossover can make it trying to separate between the two circumstances.

Misdiagnosis: Because of the side effects, people who have encountered injury might be misdiagnosed with ADHD, prompting improper treatment. Medical care suppliers need to consider an individual's set of experiences and potential injury while evaluating for ADHD.

Complex Interaction: Injury can influence mental and profound working, possibly intensifying ADHD side effects. Alternately, ADHD-related impulsivity and distractedness can expand weakness to awful encounters or the improvement of injury-related side effects.

Comorbidity: It's normal for people to have both ADHD and a past filled with injury. Tending to the two circumstances at the same time through treatment and, if fundamental, prescription, can prompt improved results.

Treatment Approach: Treatment for people with both ADHD and injury normally includes a multidisciplinary approach. This might incorporate injury-centered treatment, like EMDR (Eye Development Desensitization and Going back over), and ADHD the executives' methodologies like prescription or social treatment.

Customized Care: Every individual's involvement in ADHD and injury is exceptional. Custom-made treatment plans, created with input from emotional wellness experts, are crucial for addressing their particular necessities.

Recollect that looking for proficient assistance is urgent in understanding and dealing with these mind-boggling communications between ADHD and injury. A psychological well-being expert can give a careful assessment and prescribe suitable intercessions to help mend and work on mental prosperity.

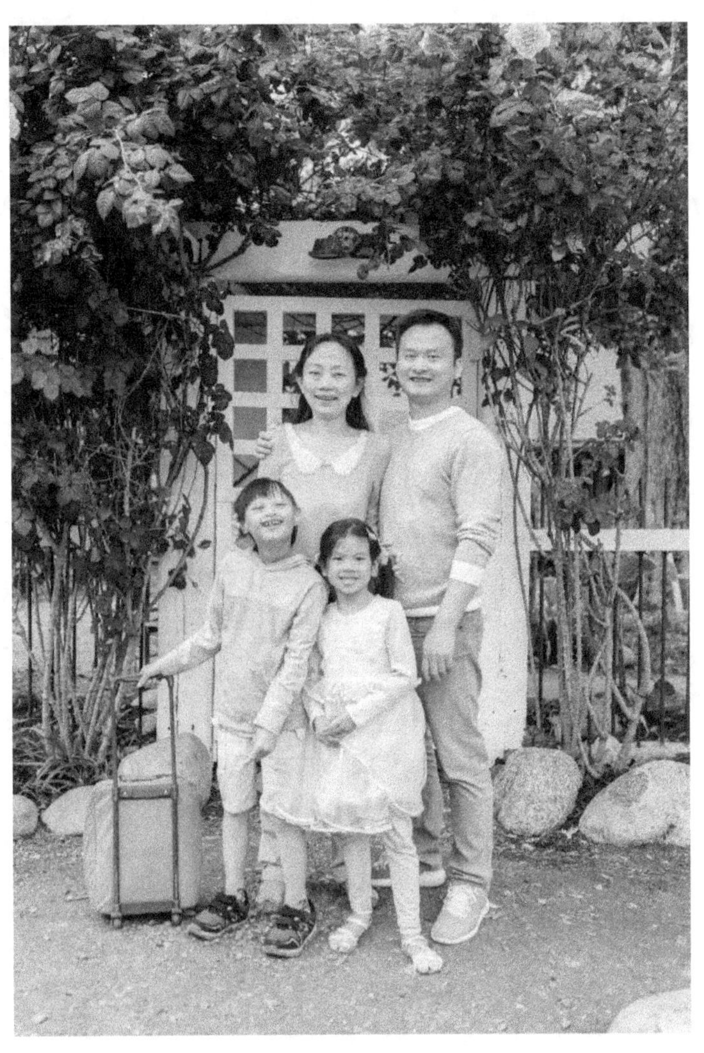

Chapter 11: Navigating the Healthcare System

Accessing ADHD Resources

To get to ADHD (Consideration Shortfall/Hyperactivity Problem) assets, think about the accompanying advances:

Counsel a Medical Care Proficient: If you suspect you or somebody you know has ADHD, begin by counseling a medical services professional like a specialist or clinician. They can give an exact conclusion and direction.

Instructive Foundations: On the off chance that you're an understudy, contact your school or college's inability administration office. They can give facilities and backing customized to your necessities.

Support Gatherings: Joining ADHD support gatherings can be useful. These can be face-to-face or online networks where you can share encounters and get counsel from others confronting comparable difficulties.

Online Assets: Investigate legitimate sites like CHADD (Youngsters and Grown-ups with Consideration Shortage/Hyperactivity Problem) and

ADDitude Magazine. They offer articles, gatherings, and assets for people with ADHD and their families.

Books and Writing: There are many books and distributions on ADHD. A few very much respected creators include Dr. Russell Barkley, Dr. Ned Hallowell, and Dr. Thomas E. Brown.

Medicine Data: If a prescription is essential for your treatment plan, talk with your medical care supplier for direction on the fitting drug and dose.

Treatment and Instructing: Social treatment and training can be viable. Consider looking for a specialist or mentor experienced in working with ADHD people.

Applications and Instruments: There are a few ADHD-centered applications and devices accessible for overseeing time, errands, and association. Models incorporate Trello, Todoist, and Focus@Will.

Government and Charitable Associations: Check with neighborhood or public government offices and philanthropic associations that have some expertise in emotional well-being and ADHD for extra assets and help.

Remain Informed: Stay up with the latest with most recent examination and improvements in ADHD treatment and the executives by following trustworthy sources and diaries.

Finding the Right Specialists

Finding the right experts for ADHD ordinarily includes talking with a medical care proficient who can give direction. Begin with your essential consideration specialist, who can refer you to experts like therapists, clinicians, or nervous system specialists experienced in ADHD analysis and treatment. It's critical to consider your particular requirements and inclinations while picking a subject matter expert.

Counsel Your Essential Consideration Doctor: Start by talking about your interests with your essential consideration specialist. They can survey your side effects, give starting directions, and refer you to trained professionals.

Therapists: Specialists are clinical specialists having some expertise in psychological well-being. They can analyze ADHD and endorse medicine if fundamental.

Analysts: Clinicians are specialists in brain research and can offer appraisals, treatment, and social mediation for ADHD.

Nervous system specialists: A few nervous system specialists have practical experience in ADHD and related neurological circumstances. They can give extensive assessments and treatment choices.

Pediatricians: If your youngster has ADHD, consider counseling a pediatrician who has some expertise in formative and social issues in kids.

Look for Proposals: Request suggestions from companions, family, or care groups who have insight into ADHD-trained professionals.

Look at Capabilities: Guarantee that the expert is authorized and has insight in diagnosing and treating ADHD.

Examination and Interview: Explore potential experts on the web and consider planning counsels to talk about their way of dealing with ADHD treatment and how agreeable you feel with them.

Protection Inclusion: Check that the expert acknowledges your health care coverage intends to limit personal expenses.

Second Sentiments: Feel free to do a subsequent assessment to investigate different treatment choices.

Recall that treatment for ADHD frequently includes a mix of treatments, including prescription, treatment, and way of life changes. Finding the right experts who comprehend your exceptional necessities is fundamental for the viable administration of ADHD.

Insurance and Financial Assistance

ADHD (Consideration Shortfall/Hyperactivity Problem) can affect different parts of life, including protection and monetary help. Here are a few focuses to consider:

Health care coverage: Most health care coverage plans cover ADHD finding and treatment, which might incorporate medicine, treatment, and specialist visits. Nonetheless, inclusion can shift, so looking into your arrangement and checking for particular necessities or limitations is fundamental.

Medicine Expenses: Some protection plans might expect earlier approval for ADHD prescriptions or have model limitations. Conventional renditions of these prescriptions are much of the time more savvy.

Treatment and Guiding: Inclusion for treatment or advising may likewise be accessible through your medical coverage, yet it can rely upon the sort of treatment and the supplier. Check with your insurance agency to grasp your choices.

Instructive Help: Kids with ADHD might be qualified for a custom curriculum administration or facilities in schools under the People with Handicaps Training Act (Thought) in the US. This can offer extra instructive help without extra expenses.

Monetary Help Projects: A few associations and establishments offer monetary help or grants to people with ADHD for different purposes, for example, instructive help or drug costs. Exploration and check whether you meet all requirements for any of these projects.

Working Environment Facilities: now and again, people with ADHD might demand work environment facilities under the Americans with Handicaps Act (ADA) to assist them with playing out their occupation.

Charge Derivations: Contingent upon your nation's duty regulations, you might be qualified for charge allowances or attributes connected with clinical costs related to ADHD finding and treatment. Counsel a duty proficient for direction.

Recall that the accessibility of protection, inclusion, and monetary help can shift by area and individual conditions.

Advocating for Your Child's Needs

Supporting for your kid's requirements in ADHD includes:

Figuring out ADHD: Find out about ADHD side effects, treatment choices, and its effect on your kid's life.

Correspondence: Keep up with open correspondence with educators, specialists, and advisors to share data and concerns.

Instructive Help: Work with schools to foster an Individualized Training Plan (IEP) or 504 arrangement to oblige your kid's necessities.

Drug The board: Whenever endorsed, screen medicine impacts and talk about any changes with the medical care supplier.

Conduct Mediations: Investigate social treatment choices and carry out procedures at home to oversee ADHD-related difficulties.

Support Gatherings: Join ADHD support gatherings to interface with different guardians confronting comparative difficulties and gain bits of knowledge.

Taking care of oneself: Deal with yourself to oversee pressure, as pushing for your youngster can interest you.

Legitimate Privileges: Know about lawful freedoms, similar to Thought, Area 504, and ADA, to guarantee your kid gets appropriate facilities.

Remain Informed: Keep awake to date with examinations and assets connected with ADHD to settle on informed choices.

Tolerance and Promotion: Keep supporting your kid's requirements after some time, adjusting methodologies as they develop and change.

Chapter 12: Supportive Therapies

Behavioral Therapy

Conduct treatment is a typical methodology for treating ADHD (Consideration Shortage/Hyperactivity Problem). It centers around assisting people with creating explicit abilities and systems to deal with their side effects. A few vital parts of conducting treatment for ADHD include:

Parent Preparing: Guardians learn strategies to deal with their kid's way of behaving, like setting clear assumptions, utilizing encouraging feedback, and giving reliable schedules.

Conduct Mediations: Specialists work with people to target explicit ways of behaving related to ADHD, similar to impulsivity or carelessness, and execute procedures to further develop them.

Token Frameworks: Token economies can be utilized to compensate for wanted ways of behaving with tokens that can be traded for honors or rewards, building up sure ways of behaving.

Self-Checking: People figure out how to follow their way of behaving and recognize examples and triggers, assisting them with acquiring more noteworthy mindfulness and control.

Interactive abilities Preparing: This assists people with ADHD in fostering better relational abilities and overseeing social circumstances all the more.

Mental Social Treatment (CBT): CBT can be adjusted to address the idea designs and inner difficulties frequently connected with ADHD.

Homeroom Intercessions: Instructors can carry out procedures to help understudies with ADHD, for example, changing the study hall climate and giving clear directions.

Conduct treatment can be exceptionally powerful, particularly when joined with different medicines like drugs.

Cognitive-behavioral therapy(CBT)

Mental social treatment (CBT) can be a useful adjunctive treatment for ADHD (Consideration Deficiency/Hyperactivity Issue). It doesn't supplant drugs, however, it can address explicit difficulties connected with ADHD. CBT for ADHD commonly centers around working on hierarchical abilities, using time productively, and motivation control through organized meetings and down-to-earth techniques. It very well may be particularly valuable when joined with different medicines, similar to prescription and conduct mediations.

Ability Building: CBT for ADHD frequently includes training people in reasonable abilities to more readily deal with their side effects. This incorporates procedures for association, arranging, and critical thinking.

Social Alteration: It can assist people with recognizing tricky ways of behaving related to ADHD, like impulsivity or distractedness, and work on procedures to adjust and further develop them.

Self-Observing: CBT might incorporate keeping diaries or utilizing applications to follow day-to-day exercises, states of mind, and ways of behaving. This self-checking assists people in turning out to be more mindful of their ADHD-related difficulties.

Objective Setting: Defining and pursuing explicit objectives is a vital part of CBT. This assists people with ADHD to stay roused and zeroed in on rolling out sure improvements in their lives.

Close to Home Guideline: CBT can likewise address personal hardships that frequently go with ADHD, like dissatisfaction and low confidence, by showing people how to deal with their feelings.

Parent Preparing: For kids with ADHD, CBT can include preparing guardians with techniques to deal with their kid's way of behaving and give an organized climate at home.

Individualized Approach: CBT is customized to the novel requirements and difficulties of every person with ADHD, making it an adaptable and versatile treatment choice.

Recall that CBT alone may not be adequate for dealing with all parts of ADHD, particularly in additional extreme cases. It's not unexpected when utilized related to different medicines, like drugs and instructive help.

Social Skills Training

Interactive abilities preparation can be advantageous for people with ADHD. It commonly centers around further developing correspondence, motivation control, and social connections. Methodologies might incorporate pretending, critical thinking works out, and rehearsing undivided attention. It's not an unexpected piece of an exhaustive treatment plan that incorporates prescription and conduct treatment. On the off chance that you or somebody you know has ADHD and is battling with interactive abilities, consider counseling a medical services professional for direction and backing.

Designated Abilities: Interactive abilities preparing can address explicit abilities like keeping in touch, alternating in discussions, perceiving expressive gestures, and overseeing hasty ways of behaving.

Organized Projects: There are organized projects and mediations intended to show these abilities. These projects frequently include bunch meetings driven by a specialist or guide.

Pretending: Pretending situations can assist people with rehearsing proper social reactions and ways of behaving in a protected climate.

Criticism and Support: Productive input and uplifting feedback are fundamental parts. People with ADHD frequently benefit from quick input to support great social decisions.

Speculation: The objective is for people to sum up these abilities to genuine circumstances. This might require progressing practice and backing.

Mindfulness: Some portion of the preparation includes expanding mindfulness of one's way of behaving and its effect on others.

Parent and Family Inclusion: Relatives may likewise be involved to help support and build up the abilities mastered during preparation.

Combination with Different Medicines: Interactive abilities preparing frequently supplements different medicines, like drug and mental conduct treatment, in overseeing ADHD side effects.

Customization: The preparation ought to be custom-made to the singular's particular requirements and difficulties connected with ADHD and social cooperation.

Recollect that the viability of interactive abilities preparation can differ from one individual to another, and it's fundamental to work intimately with medical services experts to foster an extensive therapy plan that tends to the exceptional necessities of the person with ADHD.

Parent Training Programs

Parent-preparation programs are a significant part of overseeing ADHD (Consideration Shortfall/Hyperactivity Issue) in kids. These projects furnish guardians with methodologies and abilities to help and deal with their kid's ADHD side effects. Some notable parent-preparing programs for ADHD include:

Parent-Youngster Communication Treatment (PCIT): PCIT is a proof put-together program that concentrates on further developing the parent-kid relationship and showing guardians successful conduct the board procedures.

The Unbelievable Years: This program offers nurturing classes and care groups to assist guardians with learning positive discipline methods, further develop correspondence, and diminish troublesome conduct in youngsters with ADHD.

Triple P (Positive Nurturing System): Triple P offers a scope of nurturing methodologies, from essential to more escalated, to address different conduct issues in kids, incorporating those with ADHD.

ADHD-explicit Projects: A few projects are explicitly customized for guardians of kids with ADHD, for example, "CHADD Parent to Parent" or "Adapt: Care of Guardians Enabled."

These projects commonly give training about ADHD, and conduct the executives' methods, and systems for further developing guardian-kid correspondence. They can be conveyed in social scenes, individual directing, or even through web-based assets. Guardians really should pick a program that best suits their requirements and their youngster's one-of-a-kind difficulties. Moreover, including different guardians and teachers in these projects can be valuable for an extensive way to deal with overseeing ADHD in kids.

Chapter 13: School Accommodations and IEPs

Educational Support and Accommodations

Surely! Instructive help and facilities for people with ADHD can assist them with succeeding scholastically. Here are a few normal systems:

Organized Climate: Give an organized and coordinated study hall setting to lessen interruptions and advance concentration.

Clear Guidelines: Give clear and succinct directions. Rehash significant data and utilize visual guides whenever the situation allows.

Break Undertakings into More Modest Advances: Assist understudies with separating tasks into reasonable moves toward forestalling feeling overpowered.

Additional Time: Permit additional time for finishing tasks, tests, and activities.

Incessant Breaks: Integrate brief breaks during examples or tests to take into consideration development and diminish fretfulness.

Note-Taking Help: Give duplicates of talk notes, utilization of a note-taking application, or a friend note-taker.

Visual Guides: Use visual guides, like graphs or charts, to improve learning and memory.

Elective Tasks: Offer elective tasks or evaluation techniques to oblige different learning styles.

Adaptable Seating: Consider adaptable guest plans to oblige understudies' inclinations for development or solace.

Conduct Supports: Execute the executives' systems and encourage feedback methods.

Individualized Schooling Plan (IEP) or 504 Arrangement: Foster an IEP or a 504 Arrangement to frame explicit facilities and changes custom-made to the understudy's requirements.

Prescription Administration: Work intimately with clinical experts to guarantee legitimate medicine to the board assuming it is essential for the understudy's treatment plan.

Correspondence with Guardians: Keep up with open correspondence with guardians or gatekeepers to team up on the understudy's advancement and necessities.

Recollect that each person with ADHD is extraordinary, so it's fundamental to appropriately survey their particular assets and difficulties and design facilities. The joint effort between instructors, guardians, and experts is essential to uphold understudies.

Classroom Modifications

Adjustments for understudies with ADHD in the study hall can include:

Clear schedules and timetables to give structure.

Seating nearer to the instructor to limit interruptions.

Utilization of visual guides and coordinators.

Break assignments into more modest, sensible advances.

Give successive input and uplifting feedback.

Offer open doors for development and breaks.

Limit commotion and interruptions in the study hall.

Empower association and time usage abilities.

Utilization of squirm apparatuses or stress balls to assist with the center.

Special seating away from interruptions like entryways or windows.

Carry out a pal framework for task checks and updates.

Allocate more limited, centered assignments with clear cutoff times.

Offer decisions and varieties in tasks whenever the situation allows.

Use innovation for intelligence and connecting with learning.

Give chances to visit, and brief breaks.

Speak with guardians to keep up with consistency at home and school.

Support self-checking and self-guideline methods.

Work together with custom curriculum experts for help.

Recollect that every understudy with ADHD is exceptional, so it's fundamental to tailor facilities to their particular requirements and consistently survey their advancement.

Assistive Technology

Assistive innovation can be important for people with ADHD (Consideration Shortage Hyperactivity Issue) to assist them with dealing with their everyday errands and further develop centers. A few models include:

Computerized coordinators and applications: Applications like Todoist, Trello, or Evernote can assist with tasks for the executives, planning, and setting updates.

Text-to-discourse programming: Devices like Kurzweil 3000 or Regular Peruser can change over text into expressed words, supporting understanding perception.

Voice acknowledgment programming: Programming like Winged Serpent NaturallySpeaking can be valuable for directing text, making it simpler for people with ADHD to compose or take notes.

Clamor-dropping earphones: These can assist with diminishing interruptions in loud conditions, permitting better fixation.

Center upgrading applications: Applications like Focus@Will or Brain.fm give uncommonly planned music and soundscapes to further develop fixation.

Care and reflection applications: Applications like Headspace or Quiet can assist people with ADHD to oversee pressure and further develop centers through care rehearses.

Electronic coordinators: Gadgets like smartwatches or cell phones with schedule and update capabilities can assist with monitoring arrangements and undertakings.

Computerized note taking apparatuses: Applications like OneNote or Evernote can assist with coordinating notes and thoughts carefully, making it simpler to find and audit data.

Using time effectively applications: Apparatuses like Toggl or RescueTime can help with following time spent on different undertakings and further developing time usage abilities.

Task-explicit applications: There are applications planned explicitly for overseeing ADHD, for example, ADHD Mentor and Focus@Will.

It's a memorable fundamental that the viability of assistive innovation can differ from one individual to another. It's fitting for people with ADHD to work with a medical care proficient or specialist to figure out which instruments and methodologies will be generally beneficial for their particular requirements.

Individualized Education Plans (IEPs)

Individualized Instruction Plans (IEPs) are important devices for understudies with ADHD (Consideration Deficiency Hyperactivity Issue). These plans are custom-fitted to meet the particular requirements of the understudy and may include:

Facilities: Giving facilities, for example, expanded test-taking time, special seating, or successive breaks to assist understudies with dealing with their ADHD side effects.

Conduct intercessions: Creating techniques to address incautious ways of behaving, further develop the capacity to focus, and upgrade self-guideline abilities.

Specific guidance: Offering particular guidance or intercessions, for example, mentoring or little gathering guidance, to address scholarly difficulties related to ADHD.

Support administrations: Using support administrations like advising, language instruction, or word-related treatment to assist understudies with creating social and close-to-home abilities.

Correspondence plans: Laying out clear lines of correspondence between instructors, guardians, and experts to screen headway and make fundamental acclimations to the IEP.

Objective setting: Laying out quantifiable intellectual and conduct objectives that are practical and achievable for the understudy.

The objective of an IEP for an understudy with ADHD is to establish a comprehensive and strong learning climate that boosts their true capacity and assists them with succeeding scholastically and socially. Guardians, educators, and experts must team up intently in the turn of events and execution of these plans.

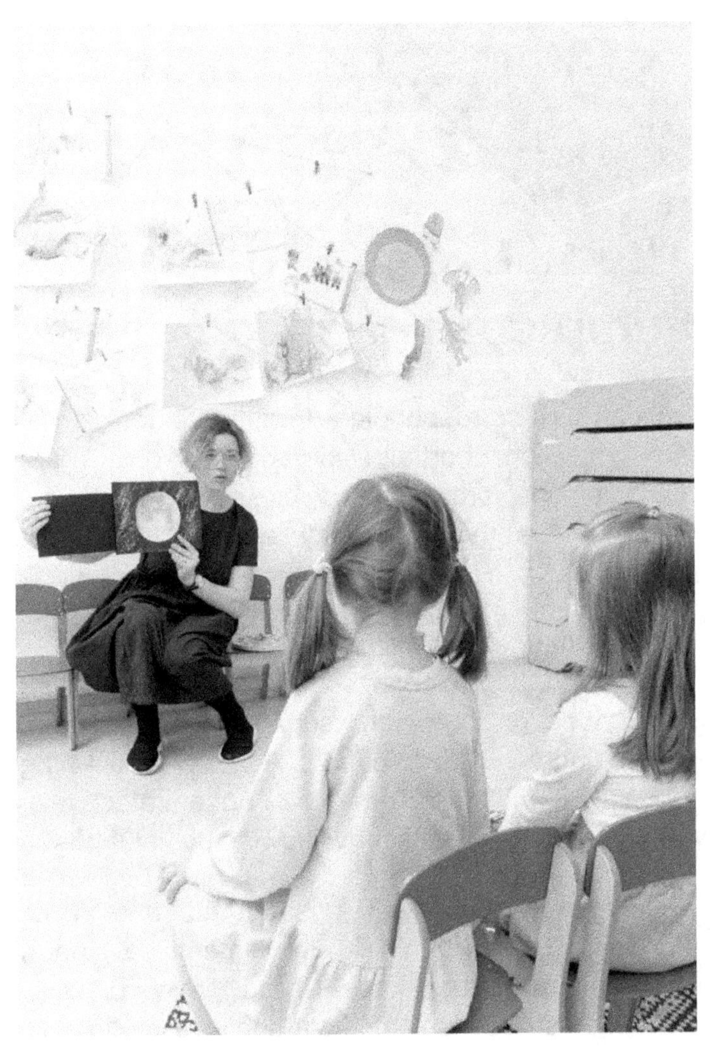

Chapter 14: Holistic Approaches

Alternative and Complementary Therapies

Option and corresponding treatments for ADHD (Consideration Shortfall Hyperactivity Problem) are much of the time utilized close by customary medicines, yet their adequacy can shift. Here are a few choices:

Dietary Changes: Certain individuals track down that wiping out specific food sources, like fake added substances or inordinate sugar, can assist with overseeing ADHD side effects. A reasonable eating regimen plentiful in omega-3 unsaturated fats, nutrients, and minerals may likewise be valuable.

Supplements: Omega-3 unsaturated fats, zinc, magnesium, and vitamin B6 supplements have been investigated for their capability to diminish ADHD side effects. Counsel medical services proficiently before utilizing supplements.

Care and Yoga: Care reflection and yoga can show unwinding and center, which might help people with ADHD.

Biofeedback: This strategy assists people with overseeing physiological cycles like pulse and mind action. Certain individuals with ADHD have tracked down it supportive in further developing consideration and self-guideline.

Neurofeedback: This type of biofeedback explicitly targets brainwave action and has been concentrated as a likely treatment for ADHD. It means to prepare people to manage their brainwaves better.

Homegrown Cures: Natural enhancements like Ginkgo biloba and St. John's Wort have been attempted, however, their viability stays unsure, and they can communicate with different prescriptions.

Needle therapy: A few people with ADHD report enhancements in concentration and smoothness after needle therapy medicines, although exploration results are blended.

Work out: Ordinary active work can assist with lightning ADHD side effects by expanding dopamine and norepinephrine levels in the cerebrum.

Conduct Treatments: Methods like Mental Social Treatment (CBT) and changing outwardly procedures can supplement medicine and show adapting abilities.

Chiropractic Care: Chiropractic changes are some of the time looked for, yet their viability in treating ADHD side effects isn't legitimate.

It's urgent to talk with a medical services professional before chasing after any other option or integral treatment for ADHD. What works can shift from one individual to another, and it's essential to have an extensive treatment plan that might incorporate a blend of treatments customized to individual necessities. Additionally, conventional medicines like prescription and conducted treatment are the most generally upheld and explored approaches for overseeing ADHD.

Yoga and Mindfulness Practices

Option and corresponding treatments for ADHD (Consideration Shortfall Hyperactivity Problem) are much of the time utilized close by customary medicines, yet their adequacy can shift. Here are a few choices:

Dietary Changes: Certain individuals track down that wiping out specific food sources, like fake added substances or inordinate sugar, can assist with overseeing ADHD side effects. A reasonable eating regimen plentiful in omega-3 unsaturated fats, nutrients, and minerals may likewise be valuable.

Supplements: Omega-3 unsaturated fats, zinc, magnesium, and vitamin B6 supplements have been investigated for their capability to diminish ADHD side effects. Counsel medical services proficiently before utilizing supplements.

Care and Yoga: Care reflection and yoga can show unwinding and center, which might help people with ADHD.

Biofeedback: This strategy assists people with overseeing physiological cycles like pulse and mind action. Certain individuals with ADHD have tracked down it supportive in further developing consideration and self-guideline.

Neurofeedback: This type of biofeedback explicitly targets brainwave action and has been concentrated as a likely treatment for ADHD. It means to prepare people to manage their brainwaves better.

Homegrown Cures: Natural enhancements like Ginkgo biloba and St. John's Wort have been attempted, however, their viability stays unsure, and they can communicate with different prescriptions.

Needle therapy: A few people with ADHD report enhancements in concentration and smoothness after needle therapy medicines, although exploration results are blended.

Work out: Ordinary active work can assist with lightning ADHD side effects by expanding dopamine and norepinephrine levels in the cerebrum.

Conduct Treatments: Methods like Mental Social Treatment (CBT) and changing outward procedures can supplement medicine and show adapting abilities.

Chiropractic Care: Chiropractic changes are some of the time looked for, yet their viability in treating ADHD side effects isn't legitimate.

It's urgent to talk with a medical services professional before chasing after any other option or integral treatment for ADHD. What works can shift from one individual to another, and it's essential to have an extensive treatment plan that might incorporate a blend of treatments customized to individual necessities. Additionally, conventional medicines like prescription and conducted treatment are the most generally upheld and explored approaches for overseeing ADHD.

Nutritional Supplements

Nourishing enhancements are not an essential treatment for ADHD (Consideration Deficiency Hyperactivity Problem). In any case, a few people with ADHD might profit from specific enhancements notwithstanding standard clinical medicines. Normal enhancements incorporate omega-3 unsaturated fats, zinc, iron, and magnesium. It's significant to counsel a medical services professional before utilizing supplements, as they can help decide whether they're fitting and safe for you or your kid. ADHD treatment commonly includes a mix of conduct treatment, drug, and way of life changes.

Omega-3 Unsaturated fats: A few examinations have recommended that omega-3 unsaturated fats, found in fish oil, may assist with decreasing ADHD side effects in certain people. They assume a part in mind well-being and capability.

Zinc: Zinc is engaged with synapse capability and may gently affect ADHD side effects. In any case, zinc enhancements ought to possibly be utilized on the off chance that a lack is affirmed through testing.

Iron: Iron lack can prompt side effects like ADHD, so rectifying a lack of iron through enhancements can be useful on the off chance that an inadequacy exists.

Magnesium: Some examination has investigated the expected advantages of magnesium supplementation in overseeing ADHD side effects, as it assumes a part in nerve capability and mind wellbeing.

Multivitamins: A decent eating routine is vital for people with ADHD. An everyday multivitamin can assist with guaranteeing they get fundamental supplements.

It's memorable fundamental that enhancements shouldn't supplant standard ADHD medicines like conduct treatment or prescription, particularly in moderate to extreme cases. Continuously talk with a medical care proficient before beginning any enhancement routine, as individual reactions can differ, and enhancements might connect with different drugs or conditions.

A balanced methodology that incorporates legitimate nourishment, normal activity, and social procedures close to clinical treatment is much of the time the best method for overseeing ADHD.

Biofeedback and Neurofeedback

Biofeedback and neurofeedback are helpful methodologies that can be used to help individuals with ADHD (Thought Inadequacy/Hyperactivity Issue). Here is a short blueprint of each:

Biofeedback: Biofeedback incorporates assessing physiological abilities like heartbeat, muscle strain, and skin conductance, and a while later giving consistent analysis to the individual. Concerning ADHD, it will in general be used to show self-rule of physiological cycles that may be associated with aftereffects, such as lessening tension or apprehension. For example, sorting out some way to control beat change can help with thought and significant rules.

Neurofeedback: Neurofeedback, on the other hand, is based on checking and giving contributions to frontal cortex activity, ordinarily through electroencephalography (EEG). Individuals with ADHD regularly show unusual brainwave plans, and neurofeedback means to set up the frontal cortex to coordinate these models. By giving visual or hear-capable signs considering brainwave activity, individuals can sort out some way to construct focus and decrease impulsivity.

Both biofeedback and neurofeedback are innocuous and can be fundamental for a total treatment plan for ADHD, habitually used and connected with various medicines and medications. Regardless, their reasonability can move to start with one individual and then onto the next, and more investigation is supposed to fathom their excessively long advantages. It's vital to talk with a clinical consideration capable who investing critical energy in ADHD to conclude whether these strategies are sensible for a particular individual.

Chapter 15: Community and Peer Support

Supportive Communities

There are a few on the web and disconnected networks that proposition support for people with ADHD (Consideration Shortage/Hyperactivity Issue). The following are a couple of choices:

Reddit ADHD Subreddit: The r/ADHD subreddit is a well-known internet-based local area where individuals with ADHD share their encounters, look for guidance and proposition support.

CHADD (Kids and Grown-ups with Consideration Shortfall/Hyperactivity Problem): CHADD is a charitable association that gives data, assets, and care groups to people and families impacted by ADHD.

ADDitude Magazine: ADDitude is a web-based asset that offers articles, online classes, and a local area discussion for individuals managing ADHD-related issues.

Nearby Care Groups: Check assuming that there are neighborhood ADHD support bunches in your space. These gatherings frequently meet face to face or basically, give a place of refuge for sharing encounters and survival techniques.

Online Gatherings: Past Reddit, you can find ADHD-centered discussions and Facebook bunches where people examine difficulties and deal with support.

Make sure to talk with medical care experts for customized direction and therapy choices.

ADHD Support Groups

ADHD support gatherings can be an important asset for people searching for understanding and direction. You can commonly track them through neighborhood psychological well-being associations, online networks, or even virtual entertainment stages. Fundamental to associate with others and share comparative encounters and difficulties to acquire backing and offer survival methods. On the off chance that you have particular inquiries or need assistance finding a care group, if it's not too much trouble, let me know.

Neighborhood Care Groups: Numerous urban communities have nearby ADHD support bunches that meet routinely. These can be found through public venues, emotional wellness centers, or by asking medical care experts for proposals.

Online Gatherings and Networks: There are various web-based discussions and networks where people with ADHD and their families share their encounters, exhortation, and backing. Sites like ADDitude and CHADD have dynamic web-based networks.

Virtual Entertainment: You can likewise find ADHD support bunches via web-based entertainment stages like Facebook and Reddit. These gatherings frequently give a space for conversations, asset sharing, and interfacing with others.

Advisor or Instructor References: Think about asking your specialist, guide, or medical care supplier for proposals on nearby or online ADHD support gatherings. They might have important bits of knowledge.

Parent Care Groups: If you're a parent of a youngster with ADHD, search for parent-explicit care groups. These can offer direction on assisting your youngster with dealing with ADHD.

School or School Assets: Instructive foundations at times have assets and care groups for understudies with ADHD. Contact the school's directing focus or custom curriculum division for data.

Recollect that the configuration and focal point of care groups can differ. Some might be general ADHD support gatherings, while others could take care of explicit socioeconomics, like grown-ups with ADHD, guardians of youngsters with ADHD, or teenagers with ADHD. It's smart to investigate various choices to track down the one that best suits your requirements and inclinations.

Peer Mentorship Programs

Peer mentorship programs for ADHD (Consideration Shortfall Hyperactivity Issue) can be exceptionally useful. These projects commonly include people with ADHD offering help, direction, and understanding to others confronting comparative difficulties. They can assist people with ADHD by:

Shared Encounters: Companion tutors can connect with the day-to-day battles of ADHD, giving a feeling of understanding and approval.

Ability Sharing: Tutors can share methods for dealing with stress, time-usage strategies, and authoritative abilities that have worked for them.

Daily encouragement: Friend coaches can offer a place of refuge to examine close-to-home and social challenges related to ADHD.

Objective Setting: They can help put forth and track objectives, encouraging a feeling of achievement.

These projects can be formal or casual and are much of the time found in schools, support gatherings, or online networks. They can be an important asset for people with ADHD looking for direction and association.

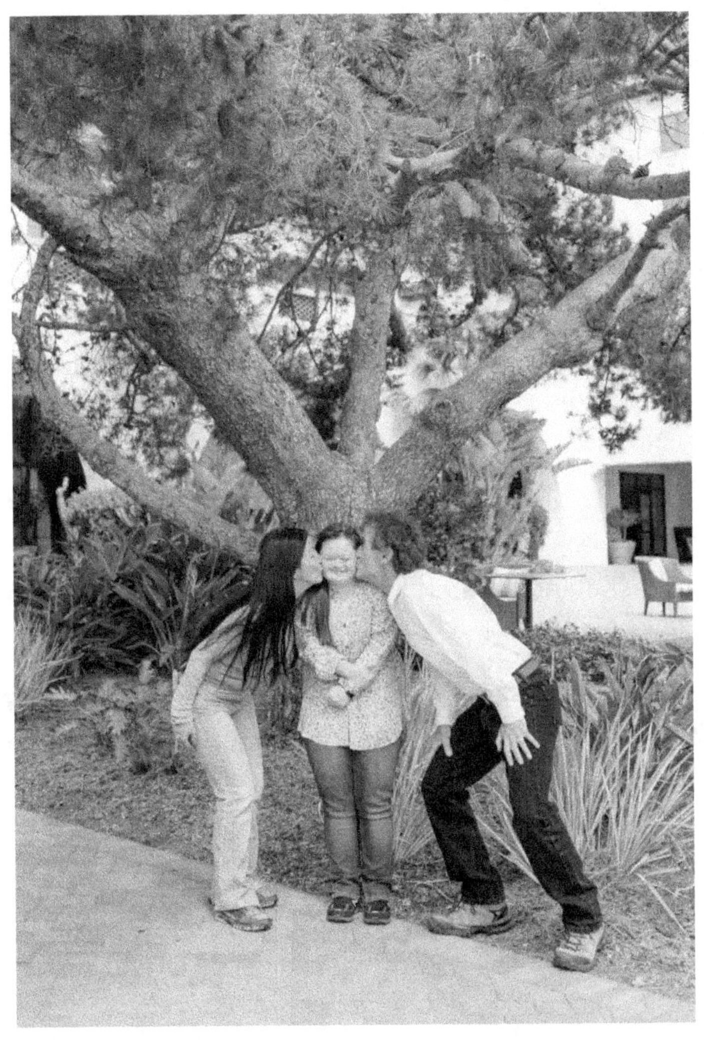

Conclusion

Nurturing the Potential in Every Child

Sustaining the possible in each kid with ADHD includes a diverse methodology that incorporates customized help, understanding, and fitting mediations. Here are a few key techniques:

Early Finding: Convenient distinguishing proof of ADHD side effects is vital. Look for proficient assessment assuming you suspect your kid might have ADHD.

Medicine The executives: A few kids with ADHD benefit from a prescription endorsed by a medical care supplier. Talk with an expert to decide whether it's reasonable for your kid.

Conduct Treatment: Social mediation, for example, mental social treatment or interactive abilities preparation, can assist kids with ADHD and foster survival methods and better self-guideline.

Individualized Training Plan (IEP): Work with teachers to make an IEP custom fitted to your kid's requirements, remembering facilities and backing administrations for school.

Organized Everyday Practice: Laying out a reliable day-to-day schedule can give strength and consistency to kids with ADHD.

Solid Way of Life: Empower customary activity, a decent eating routine, and satisfactory rest, as these variables can decidedly influence ADHD side effects.

Nurturing Methodologies: Learn powerful nurturing strategies, similar to encouraging feedback and clear correspondence, to help your kid's turn of events.

Peer Backing: Empower social association and give potential open doors to your youngster to interface with peers who figure out their difficulties.

Promotion: Be a backer for your kid's necessities, both inside the educational system and locally, to guarantee they get proper help and facilities.

Embrace Independence: Perceive and commend your youngster's special assets and gifts. Support their inclinations and interests.

Recall that each kid with ADHD is exceptional and fitting medications to their particular needs is fundamental. Look for direction from medical services experts and care groups to successfully explore this excursion.

Encouragement for Parents and Caregivers

Nurturing and providing care for a kid with ADHD can be testing, however, recall that you're making a mind-boggling showing! Your understanding, love, and backing are having a constructive outcome on their life. Commend their exceptional assets and progress, and remember to deal with yourself as well. Looking for direction from experts and care groups can be useful. You're in good company on this excursion, and your devotion is affecting your kid's life. Keep up the incredible work!